Design Controls for the Medical Device Industry

DESIGN CONTROLS FOR THE MEDICAL DEVICE INDUSTRY

MARIE B. TEIXEIRA
QA/RA Compliance Connection, Inc.
Odessa, Florida, U.S.A.

RICHARD BRADLEY
The Global Consulting Network, Inc.
Palm Harbor, Florida, U.S.A.

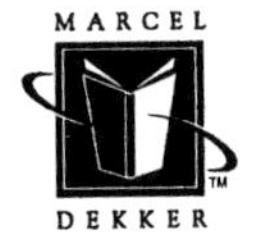

MARCEL DEKKER, INC. NEW YORK • BASEL

ISBN: 0-8247-0830-X

This book is printed on acid-free paper.

Headquarters
Marcel Dekker, Inc.
270 Madison Avenue, New York, NY 10016
tel: 212-696-9000; fax: 212-685-4540

Eastern Hemisphere Distribution
Marcel Dekker AG
Hutgasse 4, Postfach 812, CH-4001 Basel, Switzerland
tel: 41-61-260-6300; fax: 41-61-260-6333

World Wide Web
http://www.dekker.com

The publisher offers discounts on this book when ordered in bulk quantities. For more information, write to Special Sales/Professional Marketing at the headquarters address above.

Current printing (last digit):
10 9 8 7 6 5 4 3 2 1

PRINTED IN THE UNITED STATES OF AMERICA

Preface

Just what is "design control", and how did it become part of the vocabulary of the medical device industry? Simply put, design control may be thought of as a system of checks and balances that ensure that the product being developed will meet the important and essential requirements of the company developing the product. These important and essential requirements include ensuring that the product meets the needs of the end user and is safe and effective for that use. A detailed design control process was mandated for the medical device industry in the United States on June 1, 1997, when the U.S. Food and Drug Administration (FDA) mandated the design control process as part of the Quality System Regulation (QSR) for certain classes of medical devices.[1]

Before the FDA implementation, the words "design control" had provoked an emotional response from many people in the industry. People in the medical device industry viewed the concept as one more obstacle in a long list of unnecessary burdens being imposed by Washington bureaucrats. This sentiment was voiced most often in the small and early-stage medical product companies. That is not to say that the larger, and more established, medical device manufacturers were pleased with the new proposal; they simply thought of the burden in a different way. To many of these larger companies, the design control regulation was anticipated as higher overhead and subsequent lower profits. Now, several years after the initial implementation of the requirement, we need to examine whether every company affected has implemented an effective design control system and is comfortable and happy with the concept mandated by the FDA. Implemented? Probably. Are they comfortable and happy? Not likely!

In an initial survey taken between June 1997 and 1998, of 582 device manufacturers, the Center for Devices and Radiological Health (CDRH) discovered that 530 companies had implemented design control procedures. Good news! The bad news was that the survey indicated that 396 of these companies had potential design control deviations.[2] That means almost 75% of the companies surveyed had potential problems. What do these numbers really say? Are they just pointing out "learning curve" problems associated with the implementation of a new system in the industry? The answer is not clear. The

---

[1] Preproduction design controls were added to the Safe Medical Devices Act in 1990. This act gave the FDA the authority to add preproduction design controls to the cGMP regulation. This was felt necessary due to findings that showed a significant proportion, 44%, of device recalls were attributed to faulty product design. The proportion was even greater for software-related recalls at 90%.

[2] This QSIT study is available at www.fda.gov/cdrh/gmp/validationrequest.html.

high percentage of problems could also have been due to a misunderstanding by manufacturers on how to comply with the new regulations. The poor results could even have been the result of inspectors who didn't understand what may or may not have constituted compliance. However the real issue was that there was a problem.

But is there still a problem? Recently, the FDA conducted another survey of its QSIT audits.[3] Part of the survey addressed design control. In 63 audits conducted between October 1999 and May 2000, the FDA found that there were 150 design control deficiencies. The results are better than was initially seen, but there is still a noncompliance level approaching 30% in the medical device industry related to design control. There is still a problem, and there shouldn't be.

Throughout this book, we approach design control as a mandated regulation for the medical device industry in the United States. Companies that develop and manufacture class III, class II, and certain class I devices must have a design control program in place. But there is another, and in some ways more important definition of design control. Simply stated, it is a process that allows a company to make a high-quality product, from inception through production, and be reasonably sure that the resources spent in the development will result in a product that works, is useful, and is what the customer needs. What company wouldn't want to do that? Sure, lightning strikes every once in a while, but most of the very successful companies throughout the world use some form of design control to increase the odds favoring success regardless of what industry they happen to be in. This book takes those successful product development models and superimposes the FDA requirements on them to provide a blueprint for an effective and compliant design control system.

Marie B. Teixeira
Richard Bradley

---

[3] The Gray Sheet. May 10, 1999, p. 4, and June 12, 2000, p. 10.

Contents

1

Overview

AN IDEA IS BORN

If you stop to think about how much it costs to research, develop, and then manufacture a new product from the point at which somebody says it's needed to the point when the first product comes off the production line, you might wish you had a way to ensure that your new widget was the right one and it worked the first time. Think about that whole process. There are a lot of steps, and each step uses your company's most valuable resource: your people. New-product development has a voracious appetite. It consumes people, and people use time and money. Time and money are two of the things you have to keep an eye on if you want to make a profit and stay in business. An easy way to control this is to do it right the first time—and that is what design controls can help accomplish.

So what typically happens when a new product is developed, or for that matter when an old product is improved? In the ideal world, the customers say, "We want this," or "We need that and I'm willing to pay more for it." If they're not telling you that directly, then you need to go out and find out just what it is your customers really want or need. It's called *market research* and it costs money and it takes time. But if it's done correctly, you will know what kind of widget you need to develop to make a profitable sale in the first place and you won't waste time and money developing something that you know how to do but nobody wants.

ASK THE CUSTOMER

At this point, you still don't know if you can actually do what your customers want, but at least you know what you should do. Sometimes, the whole thing starts differently. Occasionally, an inventor has a great idea. It may be for something entirely new, or it may be a better way to do something that's been done before, in some way that's better than the old way. This lone inventor then sets off and begins developing the product. She risks her own money, time, and other things. One would think that this inventor might want to check to see whether anybody else thought the product was a good idea before moving ahead, but that is not often an important question for the entrepreneur*, and it's only a personal risk. Suppose, however, that your company has a department full of inventors that you call the Research & Development Department, and they come up with this really nifty idea for something new. Do you go ahead and do it because you know, or at least think, you can? Do you assume you know what's best for your customers, or do you ask them? Although the answer may seem obvious, it should be stated. You need to ask your

---

* Real entrepreneurs, please forgive us.

customers what they want, and you need to keep asking them throughout the development process and, in fact, throughout the commercial life of the product.

DESIGN CONTROLS AND THE FDA

Additionally, as the widget moves forward from idea to production, a system of checks—not only with the customer, but among the various functions of your company such as sales, QA/RA, manufacturing, engineering, R&D, marketing, and finance—needs to be implemented to ensure a high-quality product that will sell at a profit and that can be manufactured in a reproducible way. But how is this done, and how is it done in the medical device industry in a manner that accomplishes all the goals and complies with FDA regulations at the same time?

Let's start with the following question: Which medical devices are required to be developed under design controls? The FDA is clear:

> Each manufacturer of any class III or class II device, and the class I devices listed in paragraph (a)(2) of this section, shall establish and maintain procedures to control the design of the device in order to ensure that specified design requirements are met.
>
> The following class I devices are subject to design controls:
>
> i. Devices automated with computer software: and
> ii. The devices listed in the chart below:

Section	Device
868.6810	Catheter, Tracheobronchial, Suction
878.4460	Glove, Surgeon's
880.6760	Restraint, Protective
892.5650	System, Applicator, Radionuclide, Manual
892.5740	Source, Radionuclide, Teletherapy

Source: 21 CFR Part 820, Subpart C, Section 820.30(a).

Things are pretty simple at this point. Medical device manufacturers *must* institute a design control program if the device being designed is any class II or III product or a class I device identified above. So all of you making the hundreds of class I devices that can be found in the medical device industry can now close this book and move on with the other important things that you need to do to run your business.

DESIGN CONTROLS AND REALITY

Hold on a second! You're a medical device manufacturer and you would like to make a profit on what you make and the new products that you plan on making, right? Who doesn't? But you make class I devices and you're not going to do anything that you don't have to do. So if the FDA says that the new wound-dressing product line that you're developing doesn't require the process of design control, why bother? Here's why:

- Design controls help to identify what your customers want and what your competition is doing. They can even help you identify who your competition really is.
- Design controls identify inconsistencies or discrepancies in what you thought you were making when you started the development process and it identifies these problems much earlier in the process, thereby reducing the amount of redesign and rework and improving the quality of the product. Remember that the fastest way to so something right is to do it right the first time, no matter how long it takes. Besides, a well-planned design control program doesn't take all that much more time. For example, one problem notorious in all industries, including medical devices, is the invention of a product that cannot be manufactured. Using design controls can help identify, very early in a

project, any process or manufacturing problems that will occur with a newly designed product. This could save thousands of dollars and avoid unexpected delays in the project's completion.
- Once you've identified a problem, it's usually easier to fix it and adjust your limited resources early enough not to waste time and money.
- If done correctly, design controls should make conformance with all other regulatory requirements easier and simpler.
- Design controls will also make communication between departments better and ensure that the right information gets to the people responsible for other aspects of the project and therefore eventually becomes incorporated into the product that is introduced to the customer.

Our recommendation is that all medical device product developments should follow design control procedures. Well, no, not quite. Some really simple products that are classified as medical devices wouldn't gain a thing from applying all the principles of design control. On the other hand, other class I medical devices that do not *require* design control procedures would benefit from the use of design control procedures. Do you really want to launch a new wound-care line to compete with the market leaders like Smith & Nephew, Hollister, or ConvaTec without knowing whether it works or whether there are interested customers?

DESIGN CONTROLS AND THE BOTTOM LINE

The main objective of any business is to make money. The question we need to continually ask ourselves as businesspeople is whether what we are doing is moving us closer or further away from that objective. The idea that if you "build a better mousetrap, the world will beat a path to your door" is dead—

if, in fact it was ever anything more than a cute saying. Designing a new medical device requires design engineers and chemists to formulate the materials that will be used. Unfortunately, many of these otherwise bright people forget the goal of the business. They have not been hired to make the longest-lasting, strongest, most cosmetically pleasing medical device. They have been hired to make a medical device that is safe and effective for the application for which it is intended to be used. More importantly, they have been hired to do this *and* generate the most profit.

All those things like comfort, safety, effectiveness, ease of use, and durability are certainly key elements that will contribute to achieving the ultimate goal, but the prime design criterion is whether the device will make money—at least if you buy the idea that being in business has profit as its prime objective. Meeting this objective may be as simple as answering the question, "Will anybody buy this?" The product development process must also address the production, marketing, financial, and customer expectations required for the product in addition to all those things that the product must do to be safe and effective in its application. The only way to ensure that all these factors are addressed and that they do not conflict is through the creation of some sort of master plan that ensures that all aspects are being looked at and balanced in relation to each other: in other words, a design control system.

Regardless of whether the design control process is mandated by a government agency, such as it has been with medical devices, it simply makes good business sense to control what is a very expensive process. No modern company, whether large or small, can afford the experiment-till-you-drop-or-find-an-answer approach made famous by Thomas Edison. Today's world simply moves too fast and is too expensive. If your company develops and manufactures medical devices, a design control program needs to be implemented not just because the FDA has mandated it, but also because there is really no efficient alternative for directing the process of product development.

Keep in mind that the design control process does not

apply either to basic research, at least not in the context of this book, or to feasibility studies. However, once someone has decided that a particular product or design will move forward toward production, a design control process must be implemented for medical devices.

DESIGN CONTROLS AND THE CUSTOMER

The design control process is a cyclical system of checks and balances that starts and ends with the customer. Product development should start with the identification of what the customer or user wants and what he or she needs. Actually, defining the customer can be far more complicated than it seems. Is the customer the patient, the nurse, the physician, or the health-care facility? In many cases, the answer is all of these. Answering that question correctly is one of the major obstacles associated with developing a new medical device, or improving an old one. Like many developments in medical devices, the answer will likely be a combination, and maybe even a compromise, among the many requirements each wants and needs.

So now we know that if we make this device, then the nurses, doctors, and patients are going to buy it. Great start. Now what? Rush in and start doing development work? Not yet. We need a plan. The plan needs to tell us what steps must be taken in order to produce a finished product. The plan also needs to tell us who's responsible for each step, how much it will cost, how long it will take, and if we have enough of the right resources to complete the project. There are many ways to do this including simple flowcharts.

The First Law of Design Controls: Document Everything

Now all we need to do to get started is to identify what we would like the product to be or do. We need to identify all the requirements that would make this product successful:

- Who will use it?
- What are the risks?
- What kind of environment will it be used in?
- How much can it cost?
- What are the shapes, the colors, and the sizes?
- What tolerances are acceptable?
- What materials can be used?
- How should it be packaged?
- How will it function?
- How do you make a gazillion of them?
- What are the statutory and regulatory requirements?

These things are the *design inputs* from all the work that was completed prior to deciding that the development is past the exploratory or research phase and now requires design controls. These inputs may, in fact, become outputs of additional testing and design prototypes based on continued work. Remember the cyclical nature of the design control process. These and other questions are identified as the design inputs. Which of these inputs are critical and essential, which are only desires (wish lists), which can be modified, which are incomplete or vague, and which are contradictory? All this needs to be written down and dealt with—it needs to be documented.

The Second Law of Design Controls: Inputs = Outputs

Sooner or later we do some lab work and perhaps some clinical use testing on prototypes of the product and we get results and measurements from additional testing. These results are the *design outputs*. How do they compare with the design inputs? Did we meet all the goals? If not, these outputs become new inputs for subsequent tasks. Outputs also establish the acceptance criteria by which we can verify and/or validate the design. More importantly, they become the specifications, engineering drawings, quality test methods, standard operating procedures (SOPs), and manufacturing process controls of the commercial medical device. So along the way, the design team—all the people responsible for finishing the product—needs to get together on a regular basis and go over what's been done, what hasn't been done, and the results. All the information available at the time of these design review meetings is reviewed. Any inconsistencies and ambiguous or conflicting requirements need to be addressed and resolved. Any risks need to be identified, assessed, and reduced. If objective and comprehensive, these design reviews keep everything on track and prevent wasting too much time and money.

The Third Law of Design Controls: Trust but Verify and Validate Everything

Before the new product can actually get into production, we need to be sure that everything done up to this point was correct and can be reproduced time and again. We need to verify that the design criteria have been met. This verification process should confirm whether what we have accomplished (the design output) is in fact what we said we wanted to accomplish (the design input). We need to verify that we have met the acceptance criteria defined by the test methods and specifications.

Validation follows successful verification. We need to validate everything to be sure we are making what the customer asked for under actual (or simulated) production conditions. This is where we get data that says we have accomplished the developmental goal. Usually this is done through *in-vitro* performance, functional testing, and *in-vivo* clinical evaluations and trials.*

The Fourth Law of Design Controls: Transfer Is Inevitable

Once this validation is complete, it's time for one more step: the step that often causes headaches. The design and all its

* Comparison with predicate devices (form, design, function, use, etc.) and showing safety and efficacy are also considered forms of design validation.

specifications, conditions, SOPs, quality data, and drawings must be transferred to manufacturing. Manufacturing personnel need to be trained in the correct way to make the product, and everything needs to be documented, not simply because it's a requirement but because a miscommunication during the transfer can be costly and time-consuming. Product coming off the production line must meet specifications and expectations. Then, and only then, is it ready to launch.

So that's it in summary. Design controls are a simple process that ensures that what you think you are developing is what you wanted to develop in the first place and that what finally comes off the production line meets the customer's needs and expectations. The rest of this book details each step.

2

Design and Development Planning

DO WE REALLY NEED A PLAN?

Let's suppose we want to go to Paris for dinner. We decide that we really can't stay in France for too long, so we obviously need to fly. We head off to the nearest international airport and buy a ticket, get on a plane, and seven or more hours later we're in Paris ready for dinner. If that's all the planning that we've done, the likelihood that we would be in Paris having dinner is slim to none. We had the goal in mind; we wanted to have dinner in Paris. We even had a plan: Fly rather than travel by any other means of transportation. The result should have been our arrival in Paris.

The problem with this story was that we didn't have

enough information to begin with and we really didn't have a plan at all. You may think that the little story is a bit oversimplified, and it may be. But have you ever heard anybody say to you that they haven't got the time to do all that fancy planning that they do in the larger or more profitable companies? We've all heard it. It's usually followed by, "Besides, I can get the whole thing down in a few sentences."

Let's take a closer look at what really has to happen to get us to Paris for dinner. First of all, when is it we want to be there? Today? Tomorrow? Next Thursday? Easy question. We want to go tomorrow. How long are we going to stay? Now it begins to get a little more complicated. So we think about it a little and decide that we really just want to go for dinner and get back in time to watch our favorite TV show at 9 p.m. EST. That makes it a lot more difficult. But the time zones are working with us, at least on the outbound flight, and there's always the Concorde. The result now affects several other things. Does the Concorde still fly? If it doesn't, then the desired conclusion is impossible. Even if it does fly, what's the schedule? It then also becomes apparent that we just can't drive to any airport, but we need to find one of the few that the Concorde services.

So we call Air France and find out that we can get to Paris for dinner but there is no flight returning late enough (Paris time) to get us home for the TV show. We'd have to stay overnight and the best we could do is be back by noon the next day. Assuming that we have already decided that the expense of the Concorde is worth it, we now have to decide whether the added expense of a Paris hotel and other meals in Paris are affordable. Paris at night is beautiful. It's worth it. So we book the tickets. Now we have to figure out how to get to the airport from which the Concorde leaves. Not big problems, no need to discuss it; we just take care of it. Next morning we're off and are adjusting the seatbacks and tray tables for the takeoff. We're on the Concorde headed for Paris. In a few hours we'll be at the Paris airport, then to the hotel, where we'll freshen up and then head off to dinner.

Did you know that when the plane takes off and heads toward Paris, it will be off-course most of the time? If somebody doesn't do something, there is no way to guarantee that when we're ready to land we'll be anywhere near Paris. The winds encountered along the way will be enough to make a difference. But technology is wonderful; with the help of onboard computers, course adjustments are continually made and we arrive at our intended destination. Dinner was wonderful. Paris was charming. The decision to stay overnight turned out to be the best thing that could have happened.

We could have said that the first thing that needs to be done in an effective design control program is to plan. Everybody knows that, but not everybody does it. There is absolutely no way to complete a complicated project without a plan. It doesn't matter how long that planning process takes. It must be done. Just because someone can articulate the product doesn't tell you how to develop that product for manufacture and sale. If you think about the beginning of the Paris story, it may not even tell you what the product is! Remember the goal at first was dinner in Paris. The actual "product" ended up being dinner and an overnight stay.

WHAT'S A PLAN?

You can't just walk into the room where you keep your technical folks and say, "I want a new, fully functional, implantable, small intestine prosthesis." You can't wander on down the hall to the marketing folks and tell them to get ready for launch in 24 months, and then stop by the Regulatory office and tell them to file a 510(k).* We all know better: There are hundreds of things that need to happen before a product is ready for a launch. But that's why we pay all these technical, marketing, and regulatory people; they know what they have to do. But

* Everybody wants a 510(k); anything else is too much work and takes too long!

what they don't know are the details; they don't know what is happening somewhere else. And every time someone changes something, then everyone else has to adjust to what he or she is doing. Remember the wind on the way to Paris?

So, what should be in a typical plan? Plan elements vary, but in general, a plan should contain

- The goals and objectives: Define the product that is being developed.
- The organizational responsibilities: What are the interfaces between departments? How are they interrelated?
- The tasks: What are the major tasks? What tasks depend on others before they can happen?
- The resources: What will it cost? Do we have the resources (money, people, time)? If we hire two more engineers, can we do it faster?
- The time schedule: What tasks should start first? How long does each task take? What tasks can be done concurrently? Which tasks, if late, affect the outcome of the entire project (what are the critical tasks?)?
- The milestones: When do we get together to find out if there has been any progress? Are there problems? Do changes need to be made? Do major decisions need to be made? When will it end?
- The communication: How do we tell everyone who needs to know what just happened? When should major reports be issued? When do change notifications occur?

THE FDA, DESIGN CONTROLS, AND PLANS

Those are the typical elements of a project plan. There should be no surprises. So what does the FDA say it wants? The FDA says

> Each manufacturer shall establish and maintain plans that describe or reference the design and development ac-

> tivities and define responsibility for implementation. The plans shall identify and describe the interface with different groups or activities that provide, or result in, input to the design and development process. The plans shall be reviewed, updated, and approved as design and development evolves. [21CFR Part 820, Subpart C, Section 820.30(b)]

The FDA's wording is deceptively simple. The agency says you must have a plan that describes the steps of the design and development being undertaken. The first sentence of that section also says that the plan must identify the person or persons responsible for implementing the tasks. Somebody must be responsible; that's good business sense. In fact, somebody must be in charge of each step. The FDA doesn't preclude one-person companies, but this does imply a level of expertise is expected for most of the functions that are parts of a typical design and development project. Most of us wouldn't go to a bagel shop to buy an emerald ring.

The next sentence builds on this idea. The FDA requires that we identify those persons or groups that will provide the output. It doesn't matter whether those resources are employees, consultants, or other companies. Under design controls they must be identified. For example, if internal resources cannot tell you if the product you are making is sterile (assuming it has to be), then we need to find someone or someplace qualified to provide that testing. But it goes one step further; it asks that we show how all these resources will interact. Design controls require that we think about and identify how each group, sometimes working independently in their own disciplines, will be sure that what they are doing will be integrated into the tasks of what other resources are doing. The output from one group is the input for one or more other resources.

It seems obvious that different groups of people working on the same project should know what each other is doing. Everybody knows that and, for the most part, everybody does it. It's done most often with the big things, but we sometimes miss the smaller, subtle things, and most often we miss the soft requirements: the expectations and the wishes. In our experience, as both consultants and employees, the fact that one group may not know what another department or group expects is usually not due to anything sinister, but is most often due to poor communication. The folks in marketing know that the customer wants this product to be soft to the touch and have a low profile so it will be unobtrusive when worn. They've talked to users, they've run focus groups, and they made sure it was in the product development goals right from the beginning. The design folks knew about it, too. So why isn't the product being developed soft enough or unobtrusive enough for the marketing group?

Part of the reason may be a poorly written specification. Does "unobtrusive" mean a profile that's 3 cm high or 0.3 cm high? If everyone knew that it meant 0.3 cm, for example, did the design folks tell marketing (and the rest of the team for that matter) that some of the other critical objectives couldn't be met at a profile that thin? Lots of these small misunderstandings occur. Remember the greatest problem in communication is the *illusion* that it's been achieved.

So common sense and the FDA says that, "The plans shall be reviewed, updated, and approved as design and development evolves." Probably the best way to make sure this happens is to schedule these reviews on a frequent and regular basis. These meetings do more than just force a review of the project plan. They force the procrastinators to update and document what they've done, what they've discovered, and what needs to be changed and modified. It also forces other functional groups to respond to these changes and the person responsible to approve any changes or initiate a new task to resolve the fact that the input no longer quite equals the output.

PLANNING TECHNIQUES

It is beyond the scope of this book to provide an in-depth study of planning, or even some of the planning methods. But for

Task	Priority	Start date	Estimated completion date	Person responsible
Compile predicate list	A	10/1/00	10/15/00	MBT
Review R&D reports	A	10/1/00	10/15/00	ALL
Devise phase 2 clinical	A	10/15/00	10/31/00	NMcC
Verify feasibility data	A	10/15/00	12/15/00	RB

Figure 1 The action list.

technical projects several techniques have been developed and work well. They are summarized here.

The Action List

This can be made to work reasonably well for straightforward, simple product development. It is exactly what it sounds like—the good old "to-do" list. For small organizations with a simple project it can be argued that the list is sufficient. It has several shortcomings; one is that it is time-consuming to update especially when a task needs to be inserted. Figure 1 shows an action list and some of the things it should contain.

If this simple method is used to track a project, then project costs and interactions between people or other resources need to be documented separately. But perhaps the greatest problem with this method is that it gives no indication of which task should happen first or which tasks are dependent on others, and it has no predictive value. It can't tell you, once the work begins, how long it will take for the goals to be reached.

PERT

PERT is the acronym used for the planning method developed in the aircraft industry—program evaluation and review technique. It can be an extremely powerful and complex method. When it was first introduced, its power was simultaneously its most onerous characteristic. Each task is placed in a box;

inside the box is typically the starting date, the duration, and the completion date, both scheduled and actual. Other information is also included: things like the person (or group) responsible for completing the task and other resources that will be needed (including costs). The boxes are then arranged so that those that can be started simultaneously (and do not require a task to be completed before they can begin) are placed first. Other dependent tasks (those that require one of these precedent tasks to be finished) are placed on the table, and lines are drawn between the different boxes to indicate their relationships. After this is all laid out, it is relatively simple to find the longest timeline ending with the overall goal, thereby giving an estimate of the project length (and cost if you add up the dollars). This is defined as the *critical path*. It shows the tasks that need to be completed on time in order for the estimated project completion date to remain as that originally calculated. It is critical from a time point of view only. Some of the tasks on this critical path may be relatively trivial from other points of reference. Before the nice people at Microsoft, Symantec, and several other software companies large and small programmed software to automate all this, it should be apparent how difficult it was to record a change, especially if that change caused a shift in the critical path or the change required new tasks with different links.

Using one of these programs* makes the most tedious part of the plan exercise that of doing the initial plan; changes are relatively simple and automatic. These programs also allow you to add different and more detailed bits of information not envisioned in the original technique such as accruing costs, visually showing which tasks have slack time,† and leveling resources. Resource leveling (which could be done by old-fashioned brain power) allows the program to calculate the

* Microsoft Project© or Symantec's Time Line© are examples.

† The time a task can be delayed from the scheduled start time and still have no effect on the entire project.

amount of additional time it will take in order to complete tasks and the plan because one or more resources (people) have been overallocated.* Figure 2 shows the elements of a typical PERT chart.

One thing that these programs have blurred is the distinction between PERT diagrams and Gantt charts. You can switch from one to the other with the press of a button, and constructing one type automatically builds the other.

Gantt Charts

A *Gantt chart* is a graphical representation of all the tasks and milestones necessary to complete a given plan or project. The most commonly used graphical representation is a bar graph. Each task is described in a column along the left side (the y-axis) and the dates (days, months, years) from the x-axis of the chart. The bar associated with each task is proportional to the duration of the task and begins on the start date and ends on the estimated completion date. If something is late (or early), everything slides appropriately. As with PERT diagrams, Gantt charts can be constructed to show the critical path.

Most programs also plot a bar within a bar. The inside bar grows as the percentage completion of a task moves from 0% to 100%. Figure 3 shows the typical elements of a Gantt chart.

ARE PROJECTS REALLY ALWAYS LATE AND OVERBUDGET?

It seems like new-product development projects are almost always finished later, and cost more, than everyone thought they would at first. There are dozens of legitimate reasons why

---

* If your resident genius has been scheduled for three eight-hour tasks on the same day, she's been overallocated.

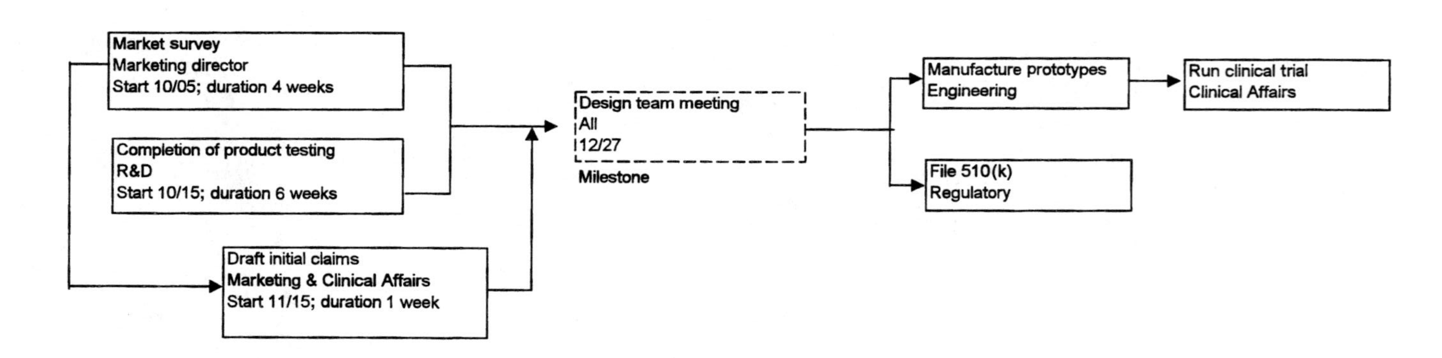

Figure 2 Simple PERT chart.

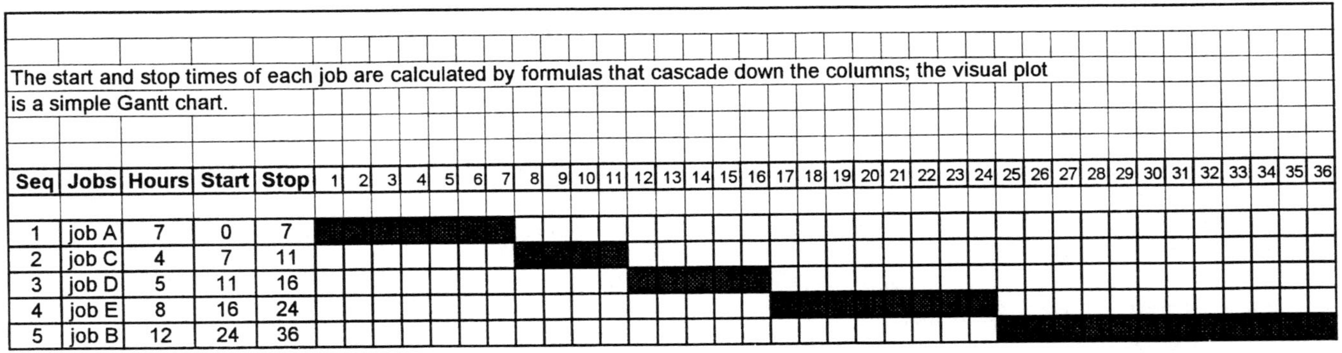

The start and stop times of each job are calculated by formulas that cascade down the columns; the visual plot is a simple Gantt chart.

Seq	Jobs	Hours	Start	Stop	1	2	3	4	5	6	7	8	9	10	11	12	13	14	15	16	17	18	19	20	21	22	23	24	25	26	27	28	29	30	31	32	33	34	35	36
1	job A	7	0	7																																				
2	job C	4	7	11																																				
3	job D	5	11	16																																				
4	job E	8	16	24																																				
5	job B	12	24	36																																				

Figure 3 A simple Gantt chart.

this could happen. Things change. The product isn't working quite the way everybody expected it to work. The competitors beat us to it and now we have to do something a little different and a little better. Reimbursement levels have changed. The product is going to cost us more to manufacture than we originally thought.

There are probably dozens of reasons that cause a development to take longer and cost more than anticipated. There are several others, however, and those are our fault. We have formulated these into the following set of rules.

The Teixeira–Bradley Rules for Ensuring a Project Will Be Completed Later Than Planned

1. If the design team consensus is that the development will take 36 months to complete, and you're the boss, insist on having it done in 18 months. Time is money, and you're the boss; they'll listen.
2. If you're a technical type like a chemist or an engineer and the marketing department asks you to develop a product that's 10 times better than the competition in performance, costs 50% less, and still has an 85% gross margin, tell them you can do it—especially if you know it's impossible, your job is not all that secure, and you're supposed to be a genius anyway.
3. If you're a marketing type, insist that the testing or quality types run that 90-day aging study quicker; show them your technical ability.
4. If you're a technical type, show them your breadth of knowledge: Point out that the sales team didn't reach the forecast first-year sales for the last product until the third year, so why should anybody rush to market with this one?
5. If you're a regulatory type, insist on adding another 6 weeks to the schedule to account for the possibility that the FDA will send the submission document

back with a number of obtuse objections. This is particularly effective if you know it's the simplest 510(k) the agency will see all year.

6. If you're a financial type, nitpick every line item in the proposed budget and hold up the project for about two weeks—just because you can.
7. If you're a quality type, insist on a 0.1 AQL for all final product testing, especially if the tests are for noncritical cosmetic properties.
8. If you're the corporate patent attorney, tell everyone that they can't do anything in public with the product until the patent has been filed and you've been waiting for two months for the engineering department to get you some drawings.
9. If you're the Vice President-in-line-to-be-the-boss, show them all your concern and agree to head a committee to decide how long each task will take. Be sure you mention that the other three members of the committee will be from a different corporate business unit.
10. If you're a human resources type, just smile and tell them that there is no way you can hire and assimilate all those new resources everyone just agreed to hire to get the project done in the shortest time.

Now, we all know that those tongue-in-cheek rules are things that *never* happen in the real world. Sure we do, just like the fact that the comic strip Dilbert® is funny because the things it shows never happen either.

One final thought about the planning process and why it often turns out that the time predictions are always faster than reality. People always underestimate; somehow they think it makes them look smarter to say something will happen faster than they know it probably will.

When assigning the duration times for the tasks, don't use the first time that came into your head. Is the time that you're thinking of the most probable time, did you account for possible unforeseen circumstances or deliveries from suppliers that might be late? Is anyone going on vacation or taking a short-term disability leave?

Try getting three different times for each task:

- The worst case, or longest time
- The most probable time, if almost everything happens correctly
- The best case, or shortest time, if everything goes right the first time

From these three numbers use a weighted average, and plug that in as the duration in your project planning—you might be surprised. Perhaps an average like:

$$\text{Most probable duration} = 2(\text{worst case time}) + 2(\text{most probable time}) + \text{best case time}/5$$

Oh, and when the president says that the project is too long—resist cutting the time estimates, at least for a while.*

* You could overestimate to begin with, or perhaps weight the average in favor of the most pessimistic time, but no one *ever* does that!

3

Design Input I

INPUT, WHO NEEDS INPUT?

Never mind who needs input. What is input? Well, for one thing, one person's input is another's output. Always keep in mind that the design control process is cyclical. Also remember that design controls begin *after* the initial exploratory phases of a project are completed.

Design controls, as mandated by the FDA and as covered in this book, do not apply to what goes on during research and during other types of feasibility studies. Before design controls can take effect in the development of a medical device, someone has to declare that the prototype, or the material sample, is likely to become a product. This declaration is usually based on feasibility testing, both laboratory and clinical use testing, that shows the product has some promise in meeting the requirements of the end user.

There also should have been a preliminary market survey that tells the company the product is worth pursuing. Someone should have also made a determination, no matter how crude, that the product could be made at a cost and sold at a price (don't forget reimbursement if it applies) that will make money. All these things become part of the design input.*

Design input is probably the most critical element of the design control process and not necessarily just from a regulatory point of view. It is certainly important to know that the medical device being developed is safe for human use and is effective for the intended use. That is, without a doubt, a regulatory issue and it is, in fact, the reason why the Pure Food and Drug Act created the FDA in the first place. But equally as important to regulatory issues is the simple fact that clearly defining design inputs is just sound business.

It is also important to want to minimize the risks where possible. No legitimate company wants to harm its customers or make a product that doesn't work. But there are other risks. A good business doesn't want to spend more money than it has, or can get, to develop a product that no one will buy. It is unimaginable that someone would waste time and money developing a product whose selling price would be 600% higher than the market will bear (or that reimbursement will allow). No one wants to develop a product that is as big as a microwave that should have been as small as a cell phone to be acceptable to doctors, nurses, and patients.† These things can be avoided with clear and accurately defined inputs.

* Of course, they are all outputs of the feasibility work. Confused yet?

† Yes we are aware that sometimes this is the only way with really new technology. Do you remember the first portable PCs from Compaq? They must have weighed 40 pounds and were bigger than many of today's desktop PCs.

THE FOUNDATION—DESIGN INPUT

Design input is arguably the most important part of the design control process. It is the foundation for the entire design and development activity. If the foundation has basic problems, then the entire structure will be suspect until those problems are identified and corrected. The inputs are the physical and performance characteristics and requirements of a device. They are the basis for the design. By spending the time and the resources to get these inputs defined accurately, a company can save an enormous amount of time and money in the long term.

Once again it is important to keep in mind the cyclic nature of the design control process. Inputs are themselves the output of previous work; they are not merely pulled out of the blue. At least they shouldn't be in an ideal world. The design inputs that begin a design control process cannot be all wishes and desires. Remember, the early exploratory work, the research, the feasibility study (whatever you would like to call it) are not part of design controls as defined by the FDA. At the point when design controls become mandatory for a medical device and this needs to be defined, hopefully you will have the output from a great deal of preliminary work. As a result, design controls should typically begin with a prototype that has been defined as likely to become a commercial medical device. The output of any testing and studies completed prior to the implementation of the design control process are the *design inputs* for the development process.

THE FDA AND DESIGN INPUT

So what does the FDA have to say about this relatively simple but extraordinarily important concept?

> Each manufacturer shall establish and maintain procedures to ensure that the design requirements re-

> lating to a device are appropriate and address the intended use of the device, including the needs of the user and the patient. The procedures shall include a mechanism for addressing incomplete, ambiguous, or conflicting requirements. The design input requirements shall be documented and shall be reviewed and approved by designated individual(s). The approval, including the date and signature of the individual(s) approving the requirements, shall be documented. [21 CFR Part 820, Subpart C, Section 820.30(c)]

This is the first time that the word "procedures" is used hand in hand with the concept of design controls. As such, look at a typical design control procedure. Such a standard operating procedure, an example of which can be found in Appendix A, fulfills the requirement to "ensure that the design requirements relating to a device are appropriate and address the intended use of the device, including the needs of the user and the patient. The procedures shall include a mechanism for addressing incomplete, ambiguous, or conflicting requirements."

THE IMPORTANCE OF DESIGN INPUT AND FDA REQUIREMENTS

As we have said, design input is the most important element of design controls. This importance is emphasized in the procedure. In addition, for complex developments, the design input phase may account for 30% or more of the entire development project! Nonetheless, some of the concepts bear repeating for emphasis in nonregulatory language.

1. Design input is the starting point and the foundation of a successful product design and development.
2. Because they are so important, design inputs need to be realistic. The critical requirements must be identified in relation to the customer (the patient and/or the user) as well as the intended use of the device.

3. The design requirements may be internally or externally imposed.
4. Design inputs include the product specifications:
   - performance characteristics
   - product description
   - safety and reliability requirements
5. Applicable statutory and regulatory requirements:
   - FDA QSR
   - ISO 9001
6. Contractual requirements:
   - special packaging
   - special storage
   - special handling and delivery
7. Environmental requirements and limitations:
   - energy—electrical, heat
   - biological—toxicity, biocompatibility
   - electromagnetic interference
   - electrostatic discharge
8. Human factors—physical characteristics and constraints:
   - intended use
   - ergonomics and ease of use
   - labeling
   - packaging
9. Design inputs need to be documented, assigned resources, reviewed and approved.
10. Ambiguous or conflicting requirements need to be resolved.
11. Finally, a designated individual(s) needs to be given the authority to sign for "approval" of the design inputs.

THE CONCEPT DOCUMENT

The *concept document*, sometimes referred to as the *product initiation request* (PIR), as it is in the example procedure in

Appendix A, is the first step along the way to an effective design control process. A model concept document is shown in Appendix B. The PIR begins to define the requirements, of the product that is, or is about to be, developed. By its very nature as a starting point it is often not comprehensive; however, it should be what its name implies—a written document. It is not a verbal agreement among a few folks to go off and develop a new medical device. In fact, even the lone inventor would benefit from producing a concept document; it would help him or her to begin to solidify that "light bulb" that went off in his or her head the day before.

Generally, the concept document is qualitative in nature, especially when being used to document a new product or application for which little is known, and when the product being developed is "new" for the company undertaking the development. It can, however, contain any known quantitative information, but that is typically left for the product performance specification (PPS) document.

In an ideal world, the marketing department of a company prepares the concept document. In an ideal world, this same marketing department is in touch with the market it serves, making this a good place to start. However, it can be initiated by anyone from any discipline; not all R&D folks and engineers are clueless.

The concept document's purpose is to broadly define the requirements of a new-product idea so that the review of whether or not that idea should be pursued can be discussed and approved by other personnel in the company. Several elements should be included in the concept document:

- A statement of purpose. Why would we want to develop this product . . . is there an opportunity? How big is the opportunity? What are we going to do?
- A statement of the market position. How is this product going to compete? Where? Against whom?
- A statement of essential or desirable characteristic.

What does the product do? What does the product need to do to be successful? What does it look like?

- A statement of the intended claims. What indications will this product be suitable for? Are there any limitations or exclusions (in demographics, for example)?
- A statement on suitable packaging. Do the intended users require special packaging for ease of opening? Does the product design require specific packaging to ensure stability?
- A statement on the clinical and technical requirements. What is the product intended to treat or manage? How is the product envisioned to provide the treatment or management? How does it differ from other similar products? How is it the same?
- What should the product cost? What does it need to cost? Will it be reimbursed?

Once this concept document is completed, and approved to move forward as an "official" development project, then a design team, composed of personnel representing different disciplines, should be assembled to prepare the product performance specification (PPS).

PRODUCT PERFORMANCE SPECIFICATION

The *product performance specification* is the last output from the research or feasibility study that was initiated by the concept document. As such this output becomes the initial input phase for the final development of the product, transfer to manufacturing, and finally release for sale.

If there has been a considerable length of time between the preparation of the concept document and the first PPS, then changes to the initial concept should be documented in this PPS. Unlike the concept document, the PPS should be comprehensive. It should also be quantitative as far as is practicable. The inputs should also be of a nature that not only can be (or have been) measured, but also can be verified. A model PPS is shown in Appendix C.

The elements that might be found in a product performance specification are

1. Performance characteristics
   - indications for use of the device
   - clinical (or use) procedures
   - relevant use settings
   - nursing home
   - acute-care hospital
   - home health care
   - hospice care
   - physician's office
   - medical specialty of the user
   - physician (specialty?)
   - registered nurse
   - medical technician
   - layperson
   - patient population—inclusion/exclusion data
   - clinical outcome analysis
2. Product characteristics
   - physical—color, dimensions, shape
   - chemical—materials used
   - biomedical/biological—maximum duration of product use *in vivo*. Reaction considerations?
   - environmental—specific storage, packaging, transportation and use conditions
   - sterilization—type of sterilant or sterilization process appropriate for the device and its package
   - packaging—a description of the specific packaging material and configuration that would be appropriate for processing, including sterilization, and ease of use by the customer
   - ergonomics/user interface—include a description of any ancillary or adjunct equipment or devices

that are necessary for the proper use of the device being developed
    - safety and reliability requirements
3. Market requirements
    - intended geographical markets
    - contractual requirements?
    - intended market segments
    - claims
    - other labeling requirements
4. Regulatory and quality assurance requirements
    - relevant regulatory requirements
    - standards and test methods

It should be obvious when these design input elements are reviewed that it is virtually impossible for a single individual, or a single department within a corporation, to effectively document the requirements. Ideally, the project team should have been consulted during the preparation of the concept document. Often that is not the case. But for the creation of the PPS the interdisciplinary team is essential to success. There are simply too many specific questions that need to be answered that require an expert in the field. If a company does not have a specific resource in-house, it needs to find an alternative. Think of the time and the money that would be wasted if a product were developed that was revolutionary for the indication but became trapped in the regulatory approval process because the developers were unaware of a certain requirement.

There are essentially three categories of design input:

1. Functional
2. Performance—both in usage and in the marketplace
3. Interfacial

Because (1) design inputs are so critical to medical device development and success, and (2) some inputs are overlooked or defined qualitatively when a quantitative measure is both desired and possible, and (3) folks often confuse necessary and critical requirements with wishes and desires, the next chapter reviews in more detail each of the typical elements/ inputs.

4

Design Input II

TO DESIGN CONTROL OR NOT TO DESIGN CONTROL

Before we look at typical design control elements in some detail, it is worth noting that some medical device manufacturers have difficulty determining when the feasibility phase or the R&D phase of a project ends and the developmental stage begins.* So perhaps we should ask, "Why does one do 're-

* Others seem to think it saves time to hold off the development phase as long as possible to avoid all the design control rules. This, of course, not only ignores the regulatory requirements but also makes little sense from the viewpoint of the effective use of resources.

search'?" Well, the first reason may be to determine the basic characteristics of a new material or a new concept. Even in industrial research, there are unknowns and certain fundamental facts that need to be studied, quantified, and explained before anyone should even think about developing a new product. Another reason for a research or feasibility stage would be to decide whether or not a business opportunity even exists. The research and development of a new product *do not* include just the technical stuff. If there is no business, there is no real product.*

So, we now enter the development stage and need to institute the design controls process as we make our first prototypes. Correct? Not necessarily. It may be quite reasonable to make several prototypes before the actual *development* begins, and sometimes before the input requirements are even partially understood. *Do not equate prototype design with finished product design*. The early prototypes lack many of the features that the final product will have. These early prototypes may not indicate a process by which they can be made; they are feasibility models. But, when there *is* enough information to think that there may be a new product or a new business opportunity, the process of design controls should be initiated by the concept document followed by the product performance specification.

PERFORMANCE CHARACTERISTICS

Since everything has to start somewhere, let's assume that the starting point for the design inputs is defining the performance characteristics of the new product being developed. This does not necessarily have to be the starting point. We could begin, for example, with the definition of the market and

---

* Of course, there are exceptions. Everyone knows that the market feasibility for the first photocopy machines showed a limited market—and now the world can't seem to live without photocopies. Stuff happens!

the needs of the patient and the end user and be just as effective.

Indications for Use

In the last chapter we list the kinds of things that help define the performance characteristics of the product. The first issue on the list is the "indications for use."

Let's use an example of a wound dressing. At this point in the development cycle, defining the indications must be more specific than saying something like, "We want to develop a wound dressing." It is simply not enough to say what the product is supposed to be or what it is supposed to do in such general terms. That is why the PPS lists this particular performance characteristic as "indications." Although the development of the product from this point might be primarily a technical and engineering function, others play an important role. Defining the indications clearly, concisely, and accurately is a necessary first step in ensuring that the needs of the market, the patient, the end user, and the regulatory environment for which the product is to be introduced are considered. Different indications may result in different functional as well as product requirements.

Suppose we say that our wound dressing should be indicated for use on chronic wounds. That's a beginning, but should there be more? Will we be marketing a product that is indicated for all chronic wounds? Will the product be indicated for leg ulcers or for bedsores, or for both? What about chronic wounds that are infected? Certainly while we're defining the indications for use, we might as well add the *contraindications* that are known. Does our research indicate there is any other type of wound that might be appropriate for the product?

Don't forget that these are inputs. They should be based on data that is relatively concrete. It doesn't mean we still can't have a wish list, but if all the fundamental work has shown that this new wound dressing does not *heal* wounds and that nothing that could be added to it would change that, then don't write the indication as "heals chronic wounds." If you did, it could set in motion a series of events that will ensure a product development that will fall short of its goals and perhaps even fail completely.

A word of caution, although it should be apparent to everyone: This section of the PPS defines the indications for use, not the *claims* for the product. The definition of the claims comes in a later section. Also remember that these are the inputs from the work that has preceded the development or are the result of the continuing work on products that are already commercialized and may have received premarket approval from the FDA.*

For example, if the inputs suggest that a wound dressing you are already marketing that is approved for chronic wounds may also be safe and effective in the management of *nonhealing surgical wounds*, a new filing to the FDA is necessary for these new indications even though the product is already "approved." It tells the regulatory people, early in the development process, that they will have to prepare the submission documentation, but only if this new indication is written into the PPS. This new indication may also signal someone in marketing of the need to come up with a new strategy.†

Clinical or Use Procedures

In the procedures section, once again based on the results of the preliminary or research work, we need to define *how* the product is to be used. We should have enough information to be fairly specific. Things may still change as the development continues, but at this point we should know how the product

---

* New indications for an "old" marketed product require a new filing.

† Think about how clever Bristol-Meyers Squibb was when they added the migraine indication to Anacin. They created a whole "new" product just by changing the box.

is to be used. In fact, it should be possible to actually write a version of the "instructions for use."*

Writing a version of the instructions for use at this point may be the best way to handle this section of the PPS. The instructions have to be written sooner or later anyway, and formatting it in this manner allows that all-important document to be reviewed, revised, and approved from the beginning.

Whether you decide to actually document this by attaching "instructions for use" or by simply listing the necessary conditions of how the product is to be used, remember that this section has several audiences. It not only tells the engineers what design parameters and requirements they need to include in the ongoing design, but it also should be written with the patient and/or end user in mind. Thus the instructions should be written in a style and with vocabulary suited for people who may not be trained in either medicine or engineering. The instructions should be kept as simple as possible even if the device is "intended for use" only by physicians. Starting early in the development cycle and constantly revising with "simple language" as a goal ensure that the instructions for use will be clear and concise by the time they are included in the commercial product.

Relevant Use Settings

Incorrectly defining the "relevant use setting" characteristic can destroy a product introduction. This particular input will have some technological and clinical facets to it, but it should be thought of as a *marketing* input. The definition may be worded by the answer to the simple question: "Where will this product most likely be used?" The answer may be deceptively simple.

* The instructions are often called the "package insert" by those who began in the pharmaceutical business.

We have the inputs of the indications for use. Where is this indication usually treated or managed? Several answers may come to mind such as hospitals, home health care, and chronic-care facilities. Depending on the device being developed, the answer may be all three. But those are just general answers and they need to be clarified and classified even further. The answer determines the likely total market for this particular product.

Where the product is to be used also helps to determine other resources. These are resources that the company may or may not have. For example, if the company has a sales force whose traditional focus is the acute-care hospital, and even more specifically only the radiography department within that acute-care setting, then it is likely that those existing salespeople will not be able to effectively sell a new product that has nursing homes as its primary sales point. This market mismatch should have been caught during the feasibility phase of the project. It is a farfetched example used only to make a point, but similar things do happen.

The dilemma may be subtler. The new product may have gone through its feasibility phase aimed all the while at the current market niche of the company. But somewhere along the way this new device was found to allow "management and treatment" in an entirely different segment of the medical industry. This could be viewed as a marketing opportunity. It could signal the start of a period of fast growth for the company as it enters a new fertile area. The one thing this new input should do is signal the fact that the corporation's resources need to be checked to be sure that they are at least adequate to perform new tasks in a new area.

Medical Specialty of the User

This should be a relatively easy input to define. Does the product require the intervention of a health-care worker, or can it be used directly by the patient? If the product, because of other characteristics, requires the intervention of a professional health-care worker, then the input should define this further. Does it require a physician, and if so should it be a physician with a particular specialty? Some devices require that the end user be a registered nurse, or perhaps a trained medical technician.

Patient Population—Inclusion/Exclusion Data

This is another characteristic that is usually relatively easy for a design team to define. Most medical devices are designed to treat or manage a specific indication, and that simultaneously defines the patient population. But its simplicity can allow the input to be misleading. For example, let's say that we are developing a device for the management of urinary incontinence. Is the patient population then all those people that suffer from any form of urinary incontinence? The answer is "probably not." First, is the device for males or females? If we continue our example by saying it's a female urinary incontinence device, then we have just cut the overall patient population by more than half. If it's an external female urinary device, it has probably cut the remaining 40% of the original total population in half again. Is the device appropriate for females with stress incontinence? The answer may lead to an even smaller fraction of the total population.

The other part of defining the patient population characteristic is defining the contraindications. Is there a group of patients in the suitable population on which the device should not be used? Is there a component or an ingredient that may cause an allergic reaction in some people? Are there situations or conditions or even other devices that interfere with the proper and safe function of the new device? Does the new device interfere with other situations in the surrounding environment? The answers to these and similar questions will help define the contraindications and therefore the ultimate patient population.

Clinical Outcome Analysis

Clinical evaluations are not required for all medical devices, but knowing the result of what will happen as the result of the use of your product is. It seems unbelievable that any company would allow the continued development and sometimes even the commercialization of a medical device without any clinical use testing at all. Because Leonardo DaVinci could envision a helicopter hundreds of years ago didn't mean that it would fly. Dozens of seemingly well-designed products have been redesigned and improved *after* simple, but objective, use tests. Even for straightforward products, a clinical use test is important. How else do you *know* that *your* product will work under the conditions it will see in use? Because a competitor's product that looks the same and has the same components has been working for years? Maybe it will work, but sometimes it doesn't.

Depending on whether any use testing was completed in the feasibility process, this characteristic may define what the product is envisioned to do and what clinical use testing needs to be done in order to verify those expectations.

This is the age of cost consciousness in the medical field. It is no longer enough to be able to manage or treat a given condition. The manufacturer must also answer "at what cost?" The answer is especially true when the selling price of the new product is higher than the currently available technology. Will it lower overall costs? What will be the outcome of using this product on the patient, on the problem being managed or treated, and on the end user's wallet?

PRODUCT CHARACTERISTICS

Physical Properties

The product's physical characteristics such as its exact dimensions, shape, and even color should be clearly and accurately defined. Everything about the physical characteristics should be clearly defined in the PPS. This includes not only the dimensions but also the allowable and acceptable tolerances. If you believe that these dimensions and tolerances are an issue only for engineering and manufacturing, think again. Ask someone with a colostomy if a pouch that is dimensioned awkwardly to the point where it is obtrusive is a good product. Don't forget that this is the section to define the different sizes the product may need to have.

Chemical Properties

The chemical properties that should be defined in the PPS include the chemical composition of all the components that make up the device. Many of today's medical devices are composed of polymers or blends of polymers, so it is important to know the nature of any additives that these polymers contain. Plastics often contain plasticizers such as oils and other materials that are used to make the materials more flexible and soft. In some polymers, notably polyvinyl chloride, or PVC, these plasticizers are often fugitive; that is, they have a tendency to migrate to the surface of the material, where they can be exposed to the patient directly.

Part of the identification of the materials that compose the product should also include identification of the interaction of these materials with other materials with which the device is likely to come into contact during normal usage. For example, manufacturing surgical gloves from a polymeric material that dissolves in alcohol or other solvents found in an operating-room setting would not be a wise idea. If the proper functioning of the device requires a material that is not included with the device—for example, "wall oxygen"—then this material should also be listed in the PPS.

Biomedical/Biological

The biomedical and biological properties of the product include several things. You must clearly define how long the product is expected to be used. This duration of use may have a two-level answer. The product may, as an example, be used to treat an indication for a 24-hour duration. It may also be used every 24 hours for 14 days. This 24-hour duration-of-use product may in fact be used to manage a chronic condition so that a single device may be used for 24 hours but changed every day for the rest of the user's life.

In this section we also need to define which body fluids and tissues the device (and each of its components) comes into contact with during normal usage. Is the device intended for use on intact skin? It is exposed to the dermal layer of the skin? Is it exposed to bone or internal tissues and organs? The answers to these questions determine the nature of the toxicity and biocompatibility testing required on the device and its components.

Environmental

The environmental property definitions include whether or not all the components of the device are suitable for operation in the working environment the device will normally encounter. In addition to that somewhat obvious definition, it is important to define the conditions for the storage, packaging, and transportation of the device, and for that matter the raw materials used to manufacture the device. This will not only aid in the determination of the shelf stability of the finished product, but also ensure that raw materials used in the manufacturing process are fresh and effective.

Sterilization

The type of sterilant or the sterilization process should be clearly defined along with a definition of what constitutes "sterile" for the product upon completion of the sterilization process. It is important that the sterilization method appropriate for the device is chosen. Several polymers, both synthetic and natural, may degrade after being exposed to ionizing radiation. In fact, although for all practical purposes there is little difference between sterilization by gamma radiation and electron-beam processing, some materials behave differently due to a dose rate effect* and therefore may limit the choice of ionizing radiation to one or the other. It would be impractical and perhaps even dangerous to use an ethylene oxide sterilization process on a material or a device that is a gas barrier. Removal of the EtO gas would be a significant problem. If the device is intended to be resterilized, the resterilization conditions and the number of cycles the device or material can withstand must be clearly understood and defined.

Packaging

A description of the specific packaging material and its configuration needs to be defined from several points of view. The package should appropriately protect the product from the environment for the duration of its useful life, including the protection of the product's sterility. It should also be designed in such a manner that would be appropriate for cost-effective manufacturing.

The packaging should also be clearly defined in terms of its ease of use for the end user or patient. A device intended for use in a sterile operating room will find few happy users if the device is difficult to remove from its package when the user wears surgical gloves. If the device's user is a paraplegic or a quadriplegic, then it is important that the package can be easily opened without necessarily requiring the assistance of another person.

Ergonomics/User Interface

This section should include a description of any ancillary or adjunct equipment or devices necessary for the proper use of the device being developed. This is especially true if they are not to be packaged with the device.†

---

* Sometimes there is a difference between delivering 25 kgy at 1 kgy per hour than delivering all 25 at one time.

† Remember to add this list to the "instructions for use."

Safety and Reliability Requirements

This section should specifically describe any conditions that will affect the safe and reliable use of the product. This may include electrostatic discharge hazards, specific voltage and grounding requirements, or protective clothing and equipment that would be recommended for use when the device is being applied, used, or removed. In addition to requirements that are related directly to the device itself, it is important to include other end user actions that may affect their safety. For example, any device that uses oxygen during its operations should take into account the standard safe use of the gas.

MARKET REQUIREMENTS

Intended Geographical Markets

This section includes the definition of the product's market in terms of geography. Is the product to be marketed and sold in the United States, European Community, Pacific Rim, and/or Asia? The answer will define not only the market size but also the regulatory requirements that must be met before the product can be introduced into a given area. It is important to involve the engineering function in this definition in order to define cultural differences that may affect the product design in different regions and countries.

Intended Market Segments

The market segment into which the device is being marketed should be clearly defined and quantified. This definition should include unit product forecasts, currency conversions, and the anticipated growth rate of the specific target market(s). For example, a wound dressing is likely to be developed and targeted at a specific wound type (e.g., surgical incisions), and perhaps even at only a fraction of that particular segment (e.g., *nonhealing* surgical incisions).

Claims

This section includes the definition of the specific claims that will be made about the device; for example, is it a therapeutic device, a patient management product? The wording of the claims should be done carefully and accurately represent any scientific and clinical findings that are known and verifiable about the device and its use in a specific indication. This section should include a review of all the other labeling related to the product such as the advertisement slicks, web site, posters, videos, and tradeshow-booth signage.

Appendix D provides a useful form for recording the claims for use with the PPS and for the design review meetings.

Other Labeling Requirements

Define any additional labeling requirements not mentioned in the other sections such as precautions and warnings. This is an ideal section for the review of photographs or line art used to show the application and function of the device being developed.

REGULATORY AND QUALITY ASSURANCE AND CONTRACTUAL REQUIREMENTS

Relevant Regulatory Requirements

This section should include all the relevant regulatory requirements that will be necessary before the device can be launched in the geographical areas noted earlier in the PPS, such as FDA QSR, EN 46001, ISO 9001, and 93/42/EEC. The section should also include the relevant standards and test methods from ASTM, ANSI, and ASQC. The AQL, sampling plans, and actual product specifications must also be included.

Contractual Requirements

These may include ISO 9000 agreements or even supply and pricing agreements with distributors, venture partners, and contract manufacturers.

5

Design Outputs

IF DESIGN CONTROLS ARE CYCLIC, WHY DIDN'T WE JUST COVER OUTPUTS?

It is true that all outputs follow inputs, which may then lead to new inputs and so on, but we have not yet really covered the concept of design outputs. Besides the overall cyclic nature of design controls, another important concept that should always be remembered is

Inputs = Outputs

What exactly does that equality mean? Look at it this way: Sooner or later the design and development activity related to a product must come to an end. If that end signaled success, then all the information and specifications that we had about the product, that is, everything the product had to do to be safe and effective and meet customer needs, should have been designed into the product. Furthermore, if successful, it was then manufactured to meet these specifications (outputs). More than that, these outputs need to be defined in such a manner that we can objectively say that they are in conformance with the inputs, that is, they must be able to be verified and validated. If these things are not true, then a risk is associated with the product and the development may not be completed—and the cycle continues.

Outputs are the work product or the "deliverable" that defines the essential and proper functioning of the device or product.

THE FDA AND DESIGN OUTPUTS

Let's see what the people at the FDA have to say about design outputs.

> Each manufacturer shall establish and maintain procedures for defining and documenting design output in terms that allow an adequate evaluation of conformance to design input requirements. Design output procedures shall contain or make reference to acceptance criteria and shall ensure that those design outputs that are essential to the proper functioning of the device are identified. Design output shall be documented, reviewed, and approved for release. The approval, including the date and signature of the individual(s) approving the output, shall be documented. [21 CFR Part 820, Subpart C, Section 820.30(d)]

There are several important requirements in that relatively small paragraph from the FDA. Among the more important are these:

1. The output procedures must define and document the methods or terms for evaluating outputs and determining their conformance in meeting the input requirements. This should be reviewed as part of the design review meetings and should be documented and maintained as part of the design history file (DHF).
2. The critical and/or essential outputs (specifications, properties) as well as the acceptance criteria must be clearly defined. These are actually the requirements for the device itself and its packaging and labeling.
3. The outputs must be approved prior to release.

The design output is the result of the effort at each design phase and at the end of the total design effort. The design outputs include the tests and procedures that may have been developed, adapted, or simply used to show conformance with the defined design inputs.

THERE MUST BE AN END

One particular characteristic of design output implied in its name is that a design and development program must come to an end sooner or later. We all assume an eventual successful conclusion to the design activities. The successful conclusion expected is that the development project will meet its goals and that the result is a safe and effective new device. Although not strictly a topic in a discussion about design controls, ending a project is an important accomplishment. In words, expressing that successful end is easy. In real life it is not often clear when a project is at an end, particularly if it has not reached the anticipated conclusion of a safe and effective product that meets *all* the design specifications. This problem is not specific to the medical device industry; it happens in any industry that develops products using an R&D and engineering department. The fault lies with several (groups of) people.

In the first instance, it is almost impossible to get a research person or an engineer to admit to either of the following:

1. That something cannot be done with just a little more work, a little more money, or a little more something.
2. That a product, especially the one being developed, could not be made a little (or a lot) better with just more time.

At the risk of irate communications from some readers, all technical people have made similar statements at least once in their careers, if not at least once during the course of every project they have worked on. Why do they do that? The answer is disarmingly simple. They do it because they really believe that virtually nothing is impossible and that things can always be made better. It would be difficult to do the job of developing in the absence of such a philosophy. They may know that in some particular case the desired outcome will not happen, but somewhere in their makeup they believe it can be done.*

The problem in a finite development situation is that resources are limited. Remember, the goal of any company is to make money. If a company is wasting money pursuing a development project that will not be achieved in a finite period of time or within a defined expenditure, it is not pursuing its goal. Countless startup companies have failed not just because they didn't know what they were doing, but because they pur-

---

* It is possible to believe that something you want to happen badly enough will happen, even though at any particular minute in time you know it won't. It is the basis of every philosophy in the world. Without a strong belief that you can accomplish what you have set out to do, or get what you want, then there is no *real* motivation to get you through the difficult periods.

sued an elusive dream and exhausted their resources. So what can be done about the problem?*

First, remember that the people charged with the development are focused on the design goals of the project; they are not focused on the resource allocation problems. Second, remember that these people are probably pretty bright. So put them in a smaller box. Remind them about the overall goal. We are not suggesting that you beat them over the head with the fact that they're spending money and time and getting nowhere (although once in a while that couldn't hurt if done correctly). What we are suggesting is that you include this "technical" group in the decision process of resource allocation. Quantify it. Is there some "rate of return" (ROR) on internal resources that you use to determine whether too much is being expended? There better be. If you're the boss and the ROR is in your head, share it! You may be pleasantly surprised. If you put an engineer or a chemist (or any bright person) in a position where he or she has to take into account that other things might be even more successful if resources were adjusted to accomplish them instead of continuing with the project he or she is working on, you might get a response that is more in touch with the reality of the business. This will allow people to reassess the probability of success of a given developmental step or, in fact, the whole development project without having to admit failure.

DESIGN OUTPUT REQUIREMENTS

As we said, design activities must come to an end one way or another. These design outputs need to be defined in such a manner that an adequate evaluation of conformance with design input requirements can be determined. They must be in

---

* This problem is by no means limited to technical people. Marketers, administrators, and professionals of nearly any discipline can be susceptible to the pursuit of the "white rabbit."

a format that can be verified and/or validated. These design outputs are *confirmed* as meeting design input requirements during design verification and validation. They are *ensured* during design review.

Design output procedures or specifications need to stipulate or refer to *acceptance criteria* and identify the critical measures/outputs for the proper functioning of the device. Critical characteristics may include special handling, storage, and/or maintenance of the device. Design outputs must also include specifications for the manufacturing process, assembly drawings, quality assurance procedures and specifications, device labeling and packaging, and the methods used for control. Design output documents need to be reviewed and approved (signature and date of approving individuals) prior to release. Finished design outputs are documented in the device master record (DMR).

Outputs typically become inputs for the next design stage. Although there may not be an output for every input, there should be an input *traceable* to each output. Remember that only approved outputs need to be maintained as part of the device history file (DHF).

Typical Design Outputs

- Product specifications
- Assembly drawings
- Component and material specifications
- Production and process specifications
- Work instructions
- Quality assurance specifications and procedures
- Packaging and labeling specifications and methods used
- Software code
- Installation and servicing procedures
- Results of risk analysis
- Biocompatibility results
- Bioburden test results
- Results of verification activities

THE DEVICE MASTER RECORD

The development project output is documented in the *device master record* (DMR). This is an extremely important document to both the FDA and the company undertaking the development. The DMR is a compilation of records that contains the procedures and specifications for a *finished* device. Note: The DMR is not a requirement of a product under development but is the record of the finished device. People have argued, based on this one word, "finished," that the DMR is one of the last steps in the developmental cycle. The argument has some validity in that things will constantly change during the development process. However, if the DMR material is compiled during the development process and revised as new information becomes available, it is less likely that important information will get lost.

In Subpart M on Records (Section 820.181), the FDA defines this important document in more detail.

> Each manufacturer shall maintain device master records (DMRs). Each manufacturer shall ensure that each DMR is prepared and approved in accordance with Sec. 820.40. The DMR for each type of device shall include, or refer to the location of, the following information:

- device specifications including appropriate drawings, composition, formulation, component specifications, and software specifications
- production process specifications including the appropriate equipment specifications, production methods, production procedures, and production environment specifications
- quality assurance procedures and specifications including acceptance criteria and the quality assurance procedures to be used
- packaging and labeling specifications, including methods and processes used
- installation, maintenance, and servicing procedures and methods

Think of it this way: If you want to tell someone exactly (1) what your product is, (2) what it is made of, (3) how to make your product correctly, (4) what equipment will be needed to do it, (5) what constitutes acceptable quality and how to test for that quality level, and (6) even how to maintain and install the proper equipment, then simply give him or her the DMR for the product. This makes the DMR one of the most proprietary files in your entire company. It essentially contains everything, even those trade secrets that allow your manufacturing process to work better than conventional processes. Treat the DMR with a high degree of confidentiality.

Remember that the DMR is not a single document, like the PIR and the PPS; it is a compilation of all documents that relate to the finished product. Take advantage of this and of the fact that the FDA allows the DMR to refer to the location of some of the contents of the DMR: Do *not* keep the entire

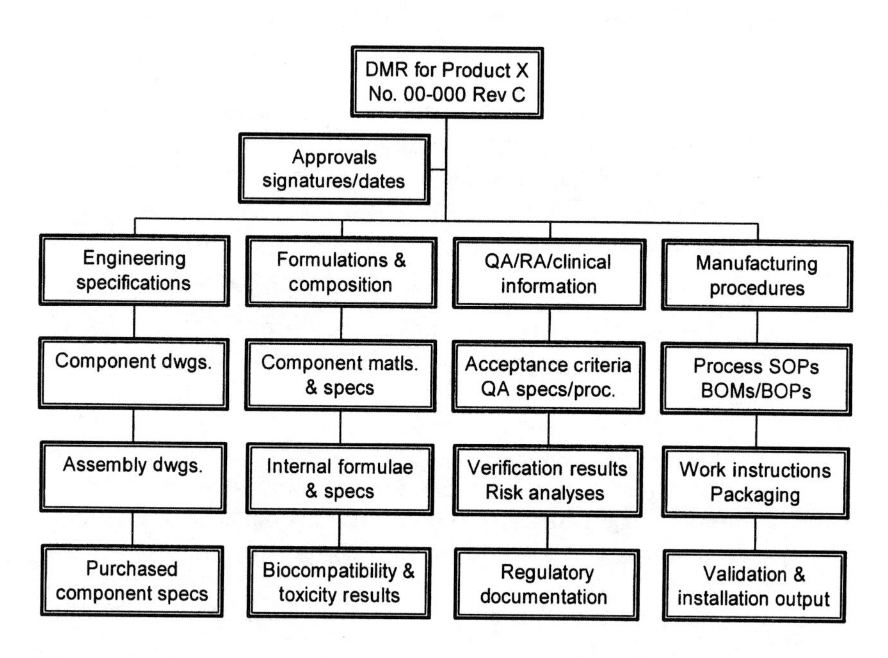

Figure 1 A generalized device master record.

record in one discrete file or location. The added work necessary to ensure that revisions to other documents and specifications are updated in the DMR file is negligible when considering the damage that can be done by fire, theft, or other catastrophic loss. Figure 1 depicts a typical device master record.

6

Design Review

NOT ANOTHER MEETING!

Although a face-to-face meeting is not a requirement, periodic design reviews are. Face it, this is American business; most of us wouldn't know what to do for a living without the occasional meeting. It is possible to have a design review without having people in the room. It could all be done, at least theoretically, by shifting reams of paper back and forth and having everybody sign off on everything, and you could always do it on the Internet, but unless at least the majority of these design review meetings are held in person, the real benefit of having them will be lost.

Remember from the beginning of this book we have mentioned two things several times. They are

- In the design controls process what goes around comes around.
- The development of a product is a team effort of people from different disciplines.

In order for everyone involved to be doing his or her "thing" correctly, each person needs to know what everyone else is doing and has done. They need to *hear* what is being said, not just see (or read) it. Design reviews should be conducted with as much personal interaction among team members as possible; otherwise things get lost in the "translation." By the time I tell another person what happened, add my little agenda, and she tells the next person, and so on, the original information is lost or distorted. People need to know as far in advance as possible what is about to happen so that if it affects their contribution to the developmental effort they can plan for the change.

THE FDA AND DESIGN REVIEWS

The FDA is clear and concise in its statement on design reviews.

> Each manufacturer shall establish and maintain procedures to ensure that formal documented reviews of the designed results are planned and conducted at appropriate stages of the device's design development. The procedures shall ensure that participants at each design review include representatives of all functions concerned with the design phase being reviewed and an individual(s) who does not have direct responsibility for the design stage being reviewed, as well as any specialists needed. The results of a design review, including the identification of the design, the date, and the individual(s) performing the review, shall be documented in the design history file (the DHF). [21 CFR Part 820, Subpart C, Section 820.0(e)]

Thus, the design review is a documented, comprehensive, and systematic examination of a product design, or design phase, in order to evaluate the adequacy of the design requirements, to assess the capability of the design to meet those requirements, and to identify problems.

Design reviews should be conducted at strategic points in the design process, which the FDA implies at the completion of certain design phases. Each review should primarily provide a careful assessment of results at that date. It should also provide feedback and information on existing or emerging problems related to the product or its development. And, like all business meetings, the design review should provide and update the team on the project's progress. It should confirm readiness to proceed to the next phase or identify the need for new tasks to be added to an action plan.

DESIGN REVIEW REQUIREMENTS

As the design is developed, it must periodically be reviewed.* Design reviews should be conducted at major decision points or milestones in the device's development cycle. These stages must be formally defined, and the timing of the design review should correspond in most cases to completion of the *milestones* of the development project plan.

The design review meeting should include representatives of all functions concerned with the design stage being reviewed. This is intended to prevent "fantasy" designs from entering production or wasting the valuable resources of a company.

Each design review needs to include an individual who is independent from the design stage being reviewed. This independent participant is necessary to bring objectivity to the

* ANSI/ASQC D1160-1995—*Formal Design Reviews* provides detailed guidance for conducting formal design reviews.

process that might otherwise be missing. In addition, other specialists in the topic being reviewed should also be present. This design review is not merely a management meeting. The specialist may have no particular management responsibilities within the company but could be a leading expert in sterilization, for example, and his or her participation could be invaluable. Design reviews must be comprehensive for the design phase being reviewed, and the participation of all these people should help to achieve this particular goal.

In addition to professional expertise in a given field, design team members should ideally possess the following qualities:

- Competency
- Objectivity
- Sensitivity

Design reviews need to include a review of verification data in order to determine whether the design outputs actually meet the functional and operational requirements. In addition, the verification data review will determine (1) if the design is compatible with all the components and any other accessories, (2) whether the safety requirements are being achieved, (3) whether the reliability and maintenance requirements are being met, and (4) if the manufacturing, installation, and servicing requirements are compatible with the design specifications.

DESIGN REVIEW FOCUS

The design review has a dual focus:

- Internal focus—feasibility of design and produceability of design
- External focus—user requirements

It may be easier to decide when a design review should be conducted if we create several somewhat artificial stages and look at what the purpose of the review would be at that point in the developmental project and some of the more important points that might be included in an agenda. The critical elements of a design review that must be kept in mind during each review are the following:

- Design evaluation
- Resolution of concerns
- Implementation of corrective actions

DESIGN REVIEW STAGES

Stage 1. Reviews Immediately After Initial Design Inputs Are Approved

The purpose of this *initial design review meeting* is to formally define and confirm the design inputs and expected outputs. *It is also used to initiate the development / manufacture phase.* The product performance specification (PPS) is a critical element of the initial design review. The initial design review meeting will also formally define the design project team. All members of the project team must be present at the initial design review meeting. Additionally, an individual who does not have direct responsibility for the design stage being reviewed needs to be present. As we have mentioned, the FDA requires the presence of specialists who are capable of providing specific expert guidance in critical areas. To review what we have said before, this initial design review may include a review of design verification data to determine (1) whether the design outputs meet the functional and operational requirements of the project, (2) whether the design is compatible with all its components, (3) whether the safety requirements are being achieved, (4) whether reliability and maintenance requirements are being met, (5) whether the labeling and other regulatory requirements have and will be met, and finally (6) whether the manufacturing process is compatible with design specifications.

A typical agenda for this initial design review might include a review of

1. The design inputs
2. The expected outputs and any known outcomes
3. The project plan
4. The risk analysis
5. The PPS
6. Any other pertinent information

Stage 2. Mid-Project Design Reviews

The objective of these mid-project design reviews is to determine whether prototypes produced by processes that are identical to (or simulate) actual production methods and procedures have performed adequately in simulated use testing and clinical evaluations.

A typical agenda for a mid-project design review might include the following:

1. Verification that the proposed design satisfies product or process requirements
2. Examination of the results of analyses, calculations, and tests
3. Evaluation of the cost-effectiveness of the product
4. Evaluation of the product performance
5. Evaluation of the manufacturability of the product

Stage 3. Final Design Review Meeting

After all verification and validation activities have been completed, a final design review meeting should be conducted. The design review should be held immediately prior to the transfer of the product to manufacturing for production. The last design review meeting is the final confirmation that the overall design output has met the overall design input. All project team members should be present at the final design review meeting. Any changes or conflicting, ambiguous, or incomplete requirements shall be documented.

A typical agenda for a final design review meeting should include:

1. A final review of the risk analysis to assess any additional real or potential hazards associated with the device under normal and fault conditions
2. Any required updates that need to be made and approved by all participating design team members
3. Any necessary changes that need to be implemented

Product/Project: Children's Swing Set

Date: April 2, 2002

Attendees: RB, MBT, NMcC, JBH

Design Phase: Midpoint

Subject: Safety concerns and assembly instructions

Minutes:

Inputs	Outputs	Review/Results	Changes
Easy-to-follow assembly instructions	Assembly instructions version 1	Difficult to follow, and parts are not identified clearly.	Add assembly drawings and a parts list.
Will not harm user	Rounded edges and safety harness	End of bolts holing the unit together are exposed and may cause injury.	Include plastic cap to cover exposed bolt ends.
For children ages 3 to 10	Must support 120 pounds	Tests verify unit will support 250 lbs. Marketing requests that one swing be designed for younger children in range.	Remove one of the three bench swings and replace with a design suitable for younger children.

Notes:

Attachments:

Figure 1 Design review meeting record.

Date of Minutes: April 2, 2002

Title of Minutes (Subject): Children's Swing Set

Check One: _______I have read and am in agreement with all aspects of the above-stated minutes.

__X__I have read and am in agreement with all aspects of the above-stated minutes with the exception of the following:

Brief Description of Discrepancy: The younger users' swing must be designed as a unit that encloses and prevents a young child from falling out during a swing arc when not being held or supported by an adult.

Signature of Team Member: JBH Date: 4/3/02

Distribution: All team members, all Department Heads, and CEO

Figure 2 Design review meeting minutes comment form.

prior to transferring the design and development specifications and procedures to production specifications and procedures

Figure 1 shows a format for recording the minutes of a design review meeting. This format allows the dissemination of the main points of the meeting to other members of the design team and to appropriate members of management. Figure 2 shows a format for members of the design team to show their agreement or disagreement with the design review minutes.

MEETING DYNAMICS

Because a successful design review depends almost as much on conducting a successful meeting as on having accurate data, it seems appropriate to review some things that we can do to ensure a successful meeting. The comments and concepts reviewed in this section are useful to all members of the design review team, including managers. They are, in fact, useful, tested, and verified concepts that will work in any business communication setting.

Communication Skills

The design review runs on information. People need clear, concise, and complete information to plan, organize, and execute their responsibilities. Whether you're leading the meeting, evaluating the outcome, or making a presentation, you will succeed or fail based on your ability to communicate. Words are the vehicles people use to communicate their goals, objectives, and performance standards. Unfortunately, many words are ambiguous and are often interpreted in different ways. The definition of what's a "good wage" may depend on whether you're paying it or receiving it. The 500 most commonly used words in the English language have an estimated 10,000 different meanings. When an engineer says, "I will complete this assignment as soon as possible," does that mean in the next two minutes, two hours, two days, or two months? We need to define our terms to make sure the receiver and sender are on the same wavelength.

Being sure that the product has "superior quality" is a great idea, but it may not explicitly communicate the desired behavior or results the team hopes to accomplish. Staff members may have their own idea of what "superior quality" means. Each person may leave the meeting ready to implement his or her own definition of "superior quality." When sending and receiving information, make sure the meaning is clear. Try saying something like, "My definition of superior quality is . . ." or "As it applies here, superior quality means . . ."

The vocabulary of product development includes many abstract ideas and concepts like "superior quality." Do not only define the terms, but also provide concrete examples to help explain the abstract idea. Examples and illustrations can provide tangible reference points to drive home the point.

Acronyms and jargon also pose potential hindrances to effective communication. In technical areas they cannot always be avoided; but because the design team is composed of people from different disciplines, be sure that acronyms and jargon are explained and clear. "The team is writing a revision to the PPS. We have new information from ASQC and ANSI that suggests this will be wise when we prepare the PMA for the CDRH." Chances are, some people will not know what all the initials mean. Spell out or define what acronyms mean, or your project may end up FUBAR.* This extra step can be the difference between understanding and confusion.

Did They Get It?

Remember, the biggest problem with communication is the *illusion* it has been achieved. Very often, defining a single word or concept is all that is needed to successfully communicate a thought or feeling. At other times verifying that someone heard what you said is prudent to ensure the message was interpreted as intended. The content and delivery of a message are obviously important, but what really counts is what the receiver heard or interpreted.

Verifying the message is a simple technique whereby the message sender asks the receiver to explain his or her interpretation of the message. If the receiver's interpretation is accurate, then a successful communication has occurred. If the interpretation is inaccurate, the sender needs to clarify and correct the misunderstanding. People are much more likely to pay attention, concentrate, and listen carefully if they know they may be called upon to give their understanding of the message. Going one extra step to check out the receiver's understanding can often save a lot of grief. If the mirrored re-

---

* For this publication that means "fouled up beyond all recognition." For a more accurate meaning, ask someone who has been in the military.

sponse is incorrect, the sender knows the message needs to be restated. Of course, some breakdowns occur simply because the listener wasn't paying attention.

The design team sits at the communication center of the development program and is particularly vulnerable to communication breakdowns. The difficulty of consistently verbalizing clear and accurate messages is immense. Never underestimate that problem. Even the most carefully worded message can be misunderstood. Periodic message verification can eliminate confusion and misunderstanding and can prevent the small and large blunders that result from communication breakdowns.

Listen and Validate

Design team members are often on the receiving end of many bits of information. It's estimated that team members spend up to 40% of their time listening. Being able to listen and accurately understand every message received is easier said than done. Listening is not easy. It requires focus, concentration, and a motivation to understand the point being made. Successful people realize that effective listening is as important as effective speaking.

How do you become an effective listener? For one thing, making eye contact with the speaker helps one to focus and concentrate. Facing the speaker puts the receiver in a good position to observe body language and other aspects of delivery. Words tell us the intellectual content of the message. Tone of voice and body language tell us the sender's emotional and energy levels. Actively observing how the message is delivered is often critical to understanding the total message.

Effective listening is an active process, not a passive one. The mind must be fully engaged when listening. No other thought should be permitted to enter your mind while listening. However, too frequently other thoughts do enter our mind and we lose focus. Some people are too busy listening to themselves to listen to someone else. Others begin to think of their response to the speaker even before they understand the speaker's point.

The best managers do not only concentrate and listen to the message; they also periodically validate their own interpretation of the message. They feed back to the speaker their understanding of what is being said. Factors like the complexity and importance of the message determine how often validation should occur. In the design review setting it should occur frequently. There are three levels of validation:

Level I: Validate by feeding back the exact words the speaker used.
Level II: Validate by feeding back a paraphrase of the message.
Level III: Validate by feeding back your interpretation of the words and body language.

Team members need to listen, not only to the words of the message but also to the tone of voice and body language. At times it's necessary to feed back what you think the sender really means but has not said. As shared understanding builds, the sender is often motivated to share additional thoughts and feelings.

Accept the Bad News

Bad news may well be the most useful information design team members receive. One common reaction to bad news is to take it out on the person delivering the message. Blaming the customer is another common response to bad news: "The product failed because they didn't follow our directions."

A third response is to deny, deny, deny.* Data indicating quality problems is criticized for being inaccurate or incomplete. Negative feedback from the customer is rationalized. All

* And if you are really adept, you follow that with counteraccusations and rationalize.

these reactions are counterproductive. The bad news can be helpful. It's a way of telling the design team that something is wrong and that a change is needed. An upset customer sends two types of messages. One has to do with the facts. The other has to do with feelings. If the team reacts defensively, and doesn't listen, there is no opportunity to improve the situation. If, on the other hand, the members listen with an open mind and acknowledge the problem, they have taken a step toward improving the situation.

Monitor and Measure

Measurements show how much progress has been made and what remains to be done. The design team's ability to measure, monitor, and control work product is directly related to the team members' ability to identify potential problems and to take corrective action if needed. Decisions based on data are a lot better than those based on speculation. Objective data removes emotion and preconceived ideas from an issue. An effective design team gets the data before making a decision. Decisions based on good data are a lot better than those based on emotions in this setting.

The team needs to draw out its members and find out who did what, where, why, and how. Separate the facts from the feelings, assumptions, and opinions. This information should be verified for accuracy with feedback received from others and from personal observations. The purpose is not to affix blame but rather to determine the facts. Given all the facts, almost anyone can make a proper decision.

Don't Confuse Motion with Progress

The design review is meant to achieve results. The results are the bottom-line measurement of performance for the design team. Activity, effort, and hard work are noteworthy factors, but the correct output is what really counts. What has been accomplished? What has been implemented? Some members of the team can project the appearance of productivity through the beehive atmosphere of activity. The atmosphere is tense, people speak rapidly, the phone rings frequently, and other employees come and go providing various input. Lots of motion, but is there any progress?

The chaos of a product development can often make it feel like a lot of work is being accomplished. Activity and effort can sometimes mislead a team into thinking goals are being met. By focusing on results, the team can ensure that activities are not ends in themselves.

The design team needs to learn a lesson from the military. A long time ago the military learned that personally going, looking, and listening are the *only* reliable feedback. A good military officer who has given an order goes out and sees for him or herself whether that order has been carried out, and how well it has been implemented.

Seeing and hearing things not only give the design team direct, unfiltered feedback; they also convey to everyone involved in the project an interest in them, their ideas, and the work they perform.

Meeting Minutes

Many design meetings end with confusion as to who has to do what and when.* During a design review meeting, as new and different action items are identified, they can be written down on a flipchart or whiteboard. The due date and person(s) responsible for each item should also be listed. At the end of the meeting, the team leader can do a quick review of all action items on the list. The team members can then leave the meeting with a clear understanding of who is responsible for which action items, and when they are due.

Making Decisions That Solve Problems

The last thing we need to discuss before returning to more information specific to design controls is decisions. Effective

* Especially when the meetings run longer than their allotted time.

design teams make decisions, from simple to complex, so it's important to know how the process works. The ability to define and solve problems leads to progress and improvement. Dealing with symptoms only wastes time, effort, and money. The process includes the following steps:

- Define the problem.
- Collect and analyze data.
- Generate alternatives, that is, brainstorm.
- Evaluate alternatives.
- Select an alternative.
- Implement the alternative.
- Evaluate the result.

In design review meetings it is imperative to identify where the project is at any given time so that a correction, if necessary, can be made.* Many problems may require multiple meetings, and different team members will frequently be at different points in the process. Little progress is made when everyone comes at a problem from a different point in the process. An effective team leader brings the group together by defining where they are in the process. Doing that improves productivity by focusing the group to concentrate on one task. Multitasking is largely a myth developed in Redmond, Washington.†

Team leaders usually prepare what they are going to say, but often they don't predetermine what questions they will ask. An important aspect of leadership is the ability to ask the right questions at the right time and to insist on answers that make sense. The answers to the right questions provide the team leader with the information he or she needs to make decisions. These questions often touch on sensitive or unpleasant topics. The questions should be simple, direct, and focused.

---

* Remember the plane on its way to Paris?

† You remember Microsoft and Windows®.

They should be framed to elicit a concrete, specific response. How the questions are asked (choice of words, tone of voice, body language) is critical. It must be done in a way that doesn't cause defensive or adversarial responses. The questions should be straightforward and asked from a neutral point of view, meaning not aggressively or with strong emotion, but not from a weak or passive position either.

Followup questions are often essential to achieve specific answers to the questions asked. If a person is unresponsive or vague, be persistent. Keep asking and probing. Rephrase the question to get to the core of the issue.

Beware of people who know the solution before they understand the problem. Some people have the tendency to go off designing systems, forms, and procedures without understanding the real problem.

Design teams are confronted with a wide range of problems ranging from broken machinery, to late deliveries, to unhappy customers, to conflicts among target properties or people. Some problems are defined in such a way that there is only one obvious solution: "The problem is that the engineers aren't working hard enough." Other problems are really symptoms of more basic underlying problems. Still other problems can be defined in such grand or global terms that it paralyzes the ability to act. In addition, design teams are often presented with problems that inspire futility. After all, if the presented problem didn't inspire futility, it would have already been solved. Right?

The hardest part of problem solving is figuring out what the real problem is. As indicated, sometimes the presented problem really isn't the problem that needs to be solved at all. Assess the accuracy of the data. Come to grips with reality, as opposed to the images and perceptions. Break through the generalizations. Complex problems should be broken down into smaller, simpler ones.

The problem statement should be free of both causes or solutions. The problem should describe what currently exists versus what is desired. The more specific and measurable the description, the better that description is. A problem statement such as, "How do we reduce the scrap rate from 5% to 3%?" provides specific and measurable criteria in the problem statement.

Once the problem is defined, the additional steps include

- Collect and analyze the data.
- Generate options or solutions.
- Evaluate those options or solutions.
- Make a decision.
- Implement that decision.
- Evaluate and measure the result to see if the problem has been solved.

7

Design Verification

WHAT IS DESIGN VERIFICATION?

Design verification provides objective evidence that design requirements have been met; if they have not been met, it shows to what extent they have or have not been achieved. It shows that the design outputs meet the design input requirements. The verification step confirms whether the outputs meet the device's functional and operational specifications. Verification is intended to show that the design is both safe and reliable and that the labeling and other regulatory requirements are satisfied. Verification answers the questions, "Did I make the product correctly, according to specifications, and can I *prove* it?"

THE FDA AND DESIGN VERIFICATION

> Each manufacturer shall establish and maintain procedures for verifying the device design. Design verification shall confirm the design output meets the design input requirements. The results of the design verification, including identification of the design, method(s), the date, and the individuals performing the verification, shall be documented in the DHF.* [21 CFR Part 820, Subpart C, Section 820.30(f)]

Of and by itself, this section really doesn't say much except that somehow we are required to verify the design being developed and document the verification, including the *method(s)* used. By insisting on the documentation of the methods used for the verification, the FDA has implied that we need to do something besides saying, "Yup, that design is what we were aiming for!" The problem is, of course, defining the word "verification." *Verification means confirmation by examination and provision of objective evidence that specific requirements have been fulfilled.*† That last sentence is the definition according to the FDA. Read it again. Sometimes you have to wonder what they were thinking when they wrote that sentence. It may have been a little clearer if it was simply stated as, "Test your design, preferably with standard methods, and document the results."

DESIGN VERIFICATION REQUIREMENTS

Procedures need to define verification methods. Any approach that establishes conformance with a design input requirement is an acceptable means of verifying the design with respect

* Design history file.

† 21 CFR Part 820, Section 820.3(aa).

to that requirement. The results of all verifications must be recorded and include identification of the design, method(s), date, and individual performing the verification. This forms part of the DHF.

TYPICAL VERIFICATION ACTIVITIES

- Design reviews
- Inspection/testing
- Biocompatibility testing
- Risk analysis
- Worst-case analysis
- Thermal analysis
- Fault tree analysis (FTA)
- FMEA
- Package integrity tests
- Bioburden tests
- Comparison to similar product designs [510(k)s]
- Measurements
- Demonstrations
- Alternative calculations
- Documentation review

The FDA likes to see verification activities shown in matrix form:

Input	Output	Result
(Requirement)	(Test method)	(Outcome = input requirement?)
Min. flow rate = 500 ml/hr	ASTM XXXX	FR ≥ = 500 ml/hr

Some typical verification examples may include the following:

Input	Output	Review/Result
Noncytotoxic	Agar diffusion method	Cytotoxicity report—Pass
Product sizes	Product specification (2 cm × 2 cm, 4 cm × 4 cm)	Inspection—Pass
Flow rate (500 ml/hr)	Test method	Test—Pass
24-hr wear time	Clinical protocol	Clinical study report
2-year expiration	Stability protocol	Stability report
CE mark	Declaration of conformity	CE technical file
Prescription	Product labeling	510(k)

RISK MANAGEMENT

Risk management is a process of applying policies and procedures to identify, analyze, control and monitor risks.* Several things need to be done to identify and manage these risks:

- Identify the risk or potential risk in the design (or the process) that may result in a hazard.
- Assign a degree or level of risk to the hazard, including the probability of its occurrence and the severity of the hazard if it occurs.
- Eliminate or reduce the problem or risk.
- Evaluate the controls and the solutions and determine whether the solution caused new problems or risks; repeat the steps if it has.
- Document the process.

Risk analysis is an important part of the overall design project and an integral part of the design controls process. A

* Design Control Guidance Document for Medical Device Manufacturers, FDA, March 11, 1997.

sample SOP for risk analysis is shown in Appendix E. In simple terms, only two outcomes are possible in the development of a medical device regardless of its specific intended use. The finished device is "safe and effective," or it is not. The FDA calls the identification and correction of use-related hazards associated with the development of a medical device human factors engineering (HFE).* The FDA has a stated goal for using HFE: "To minimize use-related hazards, assure that the intended users are able to use the devices safely and effectively throughout the product life cycle, and to facilitate review of new device submissions and design control documentation."†

So how do you do this? First, the design team needs to review all the device characteristics and determine whether they are required for the intended use and whether they could pose a real or potential hazard under normal and/or fault conditions. The team then needs to determine the degree of risk associated with the hazard. Most people have no trouble identifying the really big problems. Actually, most design engineers "design out" major hazards from the beginning. Some of the problems and risks that are often overlooked are the minor ones or those associated with fault conditions.‡ As medical device manufacturers we can't always account for every dumb or unexpected use that someone tries with a product, but we *must* try. Although these minor problems don't necessarily render the device unsafe or ineffective, they are often the difference between a good product and a great product. How many product prototypes have you seen that were intended to be placed on the human body for a couple of days and had an outline that contained right angles? Is it difficult to "round"

---

* Kay, R. and J. Crowley, Medical device use-safety: Incorporating human factors engineering into risk management, CDRH Guidance Document, July 18, 2000.

† Ibid., p. 5.

‡ Operating conditions other than "normal."

those edges and make the device a bit more comfortable for the person who will wear it?

Risk analysis is not difficult if the team remembers to think of the customers. The new-device design has accomplished all the hard stuff (like managing a fistula), but what happens to the patient when he or she puts it on? It may help manage or treat whatever problem it was intended to address, but shouldn't it be as comfortable as possible? It should also be as reliable as possible; does the design account for that? What about the needs of the physician, the nurse, or the caregiver in the home health environment? Does the device become ineffective and perhaps create a hazard for any of them? What happens to the device if it is used exactly as you intended and instructed? It should work perfectly, and most design teams think about that. What happens if someone uses the device in a manner that isn't typical? What happens if the device is used in an environment the team did not take into account? What happens when you put all these things together—the user, the environment, and the device—and they interact in a manner you didn't think of?

The reason for risk management is to answer questions such as those above. If the "hazard" created by an atypical use of a device can be reduced or eliminated in the design stage, then do it. Sometimes an identified hazard cannot be handled by changing the design. In that case it can be managed by the "warnings" and "cautions" in the labeling. A simple way to collect and document an overall risk analysis is shown in Table 1. The document is called the *risk analysis master record*. Although for space considerations it is shown here as a single-page table, it can be, and should be, an extensive and exhaustive document. Its purpose, besides the obvious documentation use, is to focus in one document all the hazards that are or could be associated with the device being developed. It implies testing and change and helps verify that the design is both safe and effective for the intended use.

Keep in mind that completing the last column "Action Taken to Reduce Risk" may entail a great deal of work and

Table 1 Risk Analysis Master Record

Product Name:		Analysis Carried Out By: Who did it? What discipline?	
Product Description: Name the specific product			
Intended Use(s): Be specific			
Characteristics could affect safety	Possible hazard associated with characteristics	Risk assessment low, medium, high	Action taken to reduce risk
1. Application: device and end user	What can happen when the device is applied?	Be objective in assigning this risk level. If it's high, say so.	Be as specific as possible and don't be limited to the space on the form. If necessary, refer to another document.
2. Materials/components used	Be specific; list all materials and any known hazard.		
3. Environmental factors	Be specific, if your device uses O_2, then keep it away from sparks or flames.		
4. Package presentation (i.e., single or multi-use)	Does the package presentation potentially cause problems?		
Evaluations for new products / complaint review for existing products		Comments	
Based on characteristics identified, and the corrections implemented, the product is considered safe for its intended use.			
Director of Quality Assurance & Regulatory Affairs	Date		

possible redesign of the product itself. This record may go on for several pages. It seems almost condescending to mention it but there are risks associated with most medical treatments and there may be risks and hazards associated with the use of a particular device. However, these major risks are almost always known to the people doing the design development and are either eliminated or minimized by the design itself or handled in the labeling if the associated risk is outweighed by the benefits delivered to the patient when using the device. Most engineers have completed a reliability analysis related to the use of a particular device. They know what will happen to the patient, the user (if other than the patient), and the surrounding environment should there be a device failure. What usually needs more attention is what will happen if someone tries an unexpected use of the product. These problems may include

- Mechanical problems—pinch points, break points, etc.
- Chemical problems—toxicity
- Biological—allergy, infection, biocompatibility issues
- Heat—burns from high temperatures in or around the device
- Electrical—shock, electromagnetic interference (EMI)
- Radiation

Remember, the team has been designing the device for use in a very particular way and most likely with a specific environment in mind, but someone could use the device in an entirely different way or in an unexpected environment. Suppose that you manufacture a skin cleanser that has been formulated into a cream. What will happen if the end user confuses the cleanser with his or her toothpaste tube and uses it to clean his or her teeth? You may not be able to prevent the occurrence, but have you done anything to minimize it?* The development team and the manufacturer both have an *obligation* to minimize risks associated with the use of the device even if, the end user uses the device inappropriately.

It should be noted at this point that this is not often easy to do, since it is sometimes considered impossible to anticipate every way that a device may be used. Even when a set of circumstances can be envisioned, it is often difficult to then esti-

* An oversimplified answer may be to design the package so that it doesn't even come close to resembling toothpaste (or denture cleaner) packaging.

mate how severe that particular hazard may be. But it must be done. The design team should:

- Take any existing information and use this information to identify use related hazards. This information can come from the anticipated use of a device and from any existing information that may be available on similar devices. In this way, hazards that may be too dangerous to actually cause to happen in a user evaluation can be addressed. There are some hazards that can actually be identified through actual or simulated use testing. If actual use testing is possible, it is preferable to use subjects that are representative of the people who will actually be using the device.
- After the information is gathered, the design team should estimate the severity of the problem; that is, the risk should be assessed.
- The team must then develop controls that will minimize or eliminate the identified hazard in the best possible manner.
- The team must now make sure that the controls implemented to control or eliminate a particular hazard have not introduced new hazards and are truly effective.
- The team should now verify that the functional and operational requirements of the device are still being met.
- Safety and efficacy should be validated.
- Finally, everything needs to be clearly and accurately documented.

HUMAN FACTORS

In its guidance document on human factors and risk management the FDA outlined the following human factors considerations for use in risk management:

- User preferences do not necessarily indicate safety and effectiveness.
- Rare and unusual scenarios resulting in serious consequences often pose the greatest threat to safe and effective device use.
- Direct inspection or paper-based analyses might not identify all hazards.
- The amount of thought that a user exerts when using the device may cause hazards during periods of high stress.
- Indicator lights, alarms, and other signals may not be appropriate in all environments. This may be especially true when there are multiple alarms on the same device.
- A device that is safe for use with one intended user may not be safe for all users. Be sure you take into account the physical and mental conditions of all possible users.
- Design the device interface to tolerate errors, and allow for backup mechanisms and systems where possible.

RISK MANAGEMENT DOCUMENTATION

As a rule, the level of documentation should be in proportion to the level of device-related hazards. In general, it should include

- The purpose and operation of the device; the patient population including those who should be excluded; a description of the device and a comparison with other similar devices if possible
- The characteristics of the user interface and any labeling
- How the user is expected to interact with the inter-

face; device maintenance and any other steps the user or patient is expected to take
- Training information for the user or patient
- Use-related hazards and their solutions
- Testing and evaluations (verification) and validation of these results

8

Design Validation

WHY VALIDATE?

Validation is necessary to demonstrate that the design is a product the marketplace needs. As a result, its purpose is to provide objective evidence that design specifications (outputs) confirm predetermined user needs and intended uses. Design validation is essentially showing by objective evidence that device specifications conform to defined user needs and the intended use(s) of the device. The design team needs to ask and answer questions such as, "Did I make the right product for the user, and can I prove it?" In terms of validation of the process used to make the device, "Does the process consistently produce a product meeting predetermined specifications, and can I prove it?" The key phrase in both of these questions is, "Can I prove it?" If you can't, your design has not been validated.

THE FDA AND VALIDATION

What does the FDA say about validation?

> Each manufacturer shall establish and maintain procedures for validating the device design. Design validation shall be performed under defined operating conditions on initial production units, lots, or batches, or their equivalents. Validation shall ensure that devices conform to defined user needs and intended uses and shall include testing of production units under actual or simulated use conditions. Design validation shall include software validation and risk analysis, where appropriate. The results of the design validation including identification of the design, method(s), the date, and the individual(s) performing the validation shall be documented in the DHF. [21 CFR Part 820, Subpart C, Section 820.30(g)]

Now don't be misled by the statement "where appropriate." As a manufacturer of a medical device regulated by the FDA, for you it is *always* appropriate unless you can document a justification for not doing it. For example, it would seem almost impossible (and foolish) to try and justify decisions made about safety without a formal risk analysis.

DESIGN VALIDATION REQUIREMENTS

Remembering that design validation can only follow successful design verification, the requirements for validation are listed below.

- Design validation must be performed under defined operating conditions. This means that the conditions under which the product is made for validation purposes, which may include clinical use tests, should be the same conditions anticipated for actual full-scale production. In general, three production runs (batches, lots, etc.) is the accepted norm.

- Validation activities must not be thought of as simply a checkmark. The chosen validation activities must provide discrete data (values or measurements).
- Validation activities must address the needs of all relevant parties (i.e., patient, health-care worker, etc.) and be performed for each intended use. If you have developed an ostomy pouch that may be used by patients with a colostomy and patients with a urinary diversion, then the clinical validation of the design must be performed on both types of subjects. Of course, reliable *in-vitro* testing could be used in place of an actual clinical trial if there is sufficient scientific and statistical evidence that the test is predictive of patient use.
- Validation activities should address the design outputs of labeling and packaging.
- Risk analysis must be *completed* in the design validation stage. If it was started during verification, then this is the phase when it should be rechecked to determine whether selected solutions to hazards actually work for the patient and the caregiver and whether the solutions themselves haven't caused additional problems.
- Software used to control manufacturing processes needs to be validated. Validation needs to start in the design phase but may finish in the production phase.
- Design validation is completed when clinical evaluation is complete. Clinical evaluation is not just a clinical trial. It may include testing for safety and effectiveness, literature searches, and 510(k)/PMA reviews.

- The results of validations must be documented and include the design method(s), date, and individual(s) performing the validation. This forms part of the design history file.
- Design validation may expose deficiencies in original assumptions (e.g., device specs/outputs) regarding user needs and intended uses. If this is true, then all discrepancies must be addressed and resolved (e.g., change in design output required or change in user need or intended use).

TYPICAL VALIDATION ACTIVITIES

Validation activities may include any or all of the following:

- Clinical studies/trials conducted through institutional review boards (IRBs) and with an investigational device exemption (IDEs). For nonsignificant risk devices an IRB approval process is usually sufficient.
- 510(k)/PMA historical database search for predicate devices.
- Stability studies on both the product and the packaging.
- Clinical evaluations in clinical or nonclinical settings (market evaluation).
- Literature search (published journal articles).
- Review of labels, labeling, packaging, and product history.
- Simulated use testing.
- Transit trials.
- Performance tests.
- Functional tests.
- Biocompatibility tests.

RISK ANALYSIS . . . ONE MORE TIME

Risk analysis, including the final identification of possible hazards associated with the design in both normal and fault conditions, must be completed in this phase of the design controls process. Any risks associated with those hazards, including those resulting from user error, should then be calculated in both normal and fault conditions. If a risk is deemed unacceptable, it must be reduced to acceptable levels by the appropriate means, which might include redesign or the addition of warnings and contraindications to the product labeling. Remember, as we have said before, *it is important to ensure that changes made to eliminate or minimize hazards have not introduced new hazards.*

COMMON RISK ANALYSIS TOOLS

In addition to the methodology mentioned in the last chapter, other risk assessment tools can be used and should be explored. These are

- FTA—fault tree analysis
- FMA—failure-mode analysis
- FMEA—failure-mode effects analysis
- FMECA—failure-mode effects criticality analysis
- HACCP—hazard analysis and critical control points*

FTA: Fault Tree Analysis

A fault tree analysis is a graphical representation of the major and critical faults associated with a design, the cause for those faults, and the potential solutions to eliminate or minimize the hazards. This tool can help identify major hazards and areas of concern in a new product design, as well as corrective actions and strategies to minimize or eliminate the problems. The nature of FTA makes it a good tool for the risk management of those devices that are less likely to cause major prob-

---

* HAACP is currently under study by the CDRH/FDA as a system to minimize the impact of the manufacturing process on product safety and performance.

lems for patients and health-care workers, that is, most class I devices.

It is relatively easy to construct an FTA:

1. Construct a box at the top of the FTA diagram. List the component to be analyzed inside the box.

2. Identify the critical hazards and faults associated with the design component. This can be done by having the group brainstorm or by creating a cause-and-effect, or "fishbone," diagram.* (A cause-and-effect diagram is explained in Appendix F.) These hazards should be placed in separate boxes below the component box being analyzed.

3. Identify the causes for each hazard or fault. These causes should be placed in ovals (or some other shape) below the fault and connected to the particular fault box with lines.

4. Work toward a controllable cause. The design team should continue working toward identifying causes until a cause that can be controlled is reached. This has sometimes been referred to as a *root cause*.

5. Identify a correction for each root cause. Upon identifying the underlying cause of a hazard, the design group can then identify corrective actions that will eliminate or minimize the problem. Boxes for each of these solutions should be drawn below the controllable cause and linked by a line.

A typical fault tree analysis document would look like Figure 1.

FMA: Failure-Mode Analysis

Failure-mode analysis is a procedure to determine which malfunction symptoms appear immediately before or after a failure of a critical parameter in the product design. After all the possible causes for each symptom are listed, the product may need to be redesigned to eliminate the problem, or other strategies may be applied to minimize the fault.

---

* The FTA can be used as a summary diagram of an FMEA. See the next section.

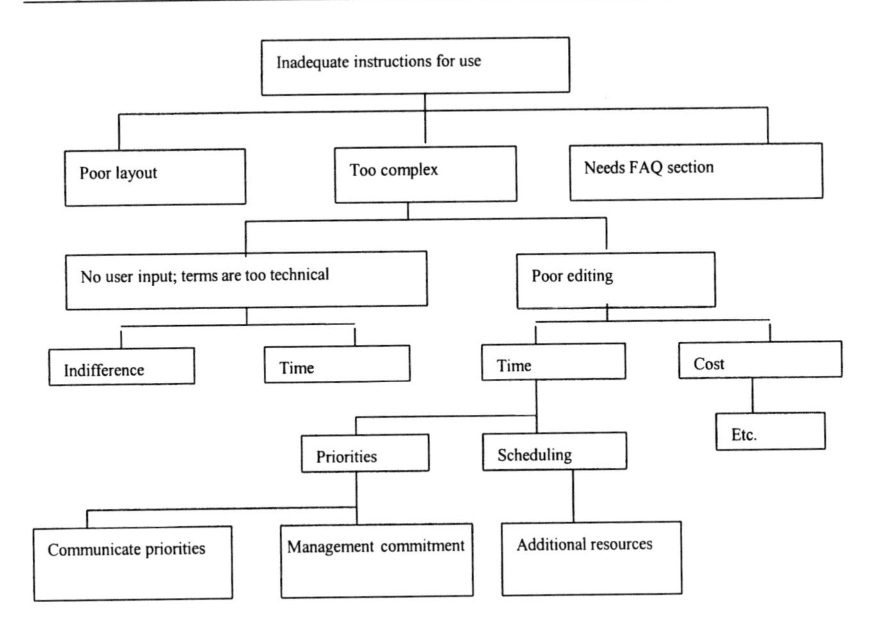

Figure 1 Fault tree diagram.

FMEA: Failure-Mode Effects Analysis

Failure-mode effects analysis is a procedure in which each potential failure mode in every component of a design is analyzed to determine its effect on other components and on the required function of the design. It can be useful in identifying critical product or process factors and designing the solutions to potential problems. It can also establish controls that may be implemented to prevent process problems and to help ensure reliability.

One method for using the FMEA analysis is to create a spreadsheet. Frequently, a multicolumn spreadsheet as shown in the Figure 2 is ideal for creating the analysis. The design team should identify all the possible modes of failure and list each of them on a separate line in column 1 of the spreadsheet (Mode of failure). The team can then create a list of the possible causes for each of the failures and list each

Failure mode	Cause of failure	Failure effect	Frequency of occurrence	Severity	Chance of detection	Risk factor	Action	Design validation
Device not installed properly	Inexperienced installer	Device must be reinstalled	1	8	10	80	Train installers	Training records
	Customer requirements not clear	Device failure	7	8	9	504	Edit installation instructions	Installation SOP
Device components detach during use	Assembly of device is incorrect	Device failure	3	10	10	300	Review assembly SOP Review inspection tests	SOP review and process validation Review test methods and AQL
	Use environment is not appropriate	Device failure	1	10	10	100	Failure test for environmental factors	Revise labeling
	Inappropriate material used to join components	Device failure	5	10	10	500	Test component attachment strength	Test report

Figure 2 FMEA chart.

cause in column 2 (Cause of failure). Column 3 could be used to list the impact of the failures on the customer, the product, or the process (Failure effect). In columns 4 to 6 a table of relative values* is assigned for each failure with regard to frequency of occurrence, impact on the customer, and likelihood of detection. These values, which the consensus of the team

* On a scale of 1 to 10, a 1 would indicate a frequency of less than 2 and a 10 would indicate a frequency of greater than 25. Using the same scale for "severity" a score of 1 indicates a trivial problem, a 10 indicates loss of the customer, and a 5 might indicate a formal complaint. For "detection" a 1 would indicate certain detection while a 10 would indicate there was no possible way to predict the problem would occur.

(or actual data) determines, are placed in the appropriate spreadsheet cell. A risk factor is then calculated by multiplying the values in each row of columns 4, 5, and 6. This risk factor is recorded in the next column of the spreadsheet. The remedy is then recorded in column 7 (Design action), and the method for verifying that the action has been accomplished is shown in column 8.

FMECA: Failure-Mode Effects and Criticality Analysis

Failure-mode effects and criticality analysis is a procedure performed with an FMEA analysis to classify each potential failure relative to a list of critical factors and helps determine what function (or resource) is responsible for the critical factors.

A spreadsheet method is also useful for preparing the criticality analysis. Once again, a multicolumn spreadsheet is created. Column 1 of the spreadsheet is used to identify the features and/or components, and all the remaining columns are used to identify the critical factors. The features or components of the device are listed in the first column. The critical factors for each of these features are then listed in the appropriate row. The number of columns of the spreadsheet depends upon the critical factors identified. A value of high (H), medium (M), or low (L) representing the risk associated with each feature is placed in the appropriate cell of the spreadsheet. The lower portion of the spreadsheet is used to indicate which internal function or other resource controls is responsible for a particular factor. Figure 3 shows a criticality analysis spreadsheet.

HACCP: Hazard Analysis and Critical Control Points

The FDA has begun a feasibility study to determine if HACCP can help the CDRH in

Features/ components	Availability of manufacturing & eng. input	Technical writer availability	Quality assurance input	Process validation
Engineering pilot runs	H		H	L
Manufacturing feedback	H		H	
Recommendations	H	M	H	H
Draft completed		H		
Responsible group				
Manufacturing	X			
QA			X	
Documentation group		X		
Engineering group	X			X

Figure 3 Criticality analysis, manufacturing process (example).

1. Premarket submissions in both the product and process review
2. Identifying and correcting problems for devices currently on the market that have performance issues
3. Streamlining premarket inspections

According to the FDA, the key elements of the system include

- Identification of all potential hazards to safety and performance for both the product and the process
- Identification of the corresponding corrective actions for the identified hazards
- Identification and control of the hazards at critical steps during the manufacturing process, the so-called critical control points
- Documentation that this control is maintained on an ongoing basis

It is believed that this system will identify hazards more quickly and specifically and allow preventative measures to be taken sooner, thereby reducing reliance on government inspection. Because it is a well-known fact that you cannot inspect quality into a product, that is a belief with which it is difficult to argue.*

RISK ASSESSMENT OF MEDICAL DEVICE MATERIALS

The principles of risk management mentioned in the previous sections also apply to the materials used as or in medical devices. A number of other things should be explored when evaluating materials.† Questions need to be answered when selecting a material for use as or in a medical device. These questions include

How will the material be exposed to the patient, and for how long? For example, the material (or the device) may be in contact with a patient for only a few minutes or an hour. Some materials may be in contact with a patient for 24 hours and may be used for only a matter of days or for the rest of the patient's life.

Will the material be in contact with intact skin? Blood? Internal organs? It seems fairly obvious that applications that will contain materials that will always be in contact with intact skin need a different level of evaluation than a material that may be in contact with the blood supply or an internal organ.

---

* As the FDA has not yet adopted HACCP, the methodology is not included. Information about the program can be obtained from the FDA by contacting Adrianne Galdi, the team leader for the study at the CDRH.

† These are preferably evaluated at the beginning of the material selection process.

Is the material stable in the environment intended for use? Will other chemicals or materials used in the treatment setting cause the material to change? Even for simple materials this can be a difficult question to answer, as it is often difficult to predict the environment in which the end user will ultimately use the material. This is the reason for the risk assessment. A lot is known about materials and their stability under a wide variety of conditions. Even if it seems impossible that your material or device could not possibly encounter adverse conditions, they should be evaluated and assessed. Under some circumstances, perhaps the best you can do is to warn potential users of unsafe environmental conditions and put that warning in the product labeling.

Will other materials or conditions cause the material to leach some of its components? Strictly speaking, this question may be part of the environmental considerations of a material. However, some polymeric materials are themselves a physical blend of a variety of other materials used to impart specific properties to the finished entity. These properties might include flexibility, specific adherence, absorption, color, and any number of other things. Many of the ingredients used to make these property modifications are not polymers themselves but are relatively low-molecular-weight materials. Low-molecular-weight materials often migrate to the surface of the polymer that forms the matrix. Temperature, pressure, and contact with other materials can cause this migration to occur faster. Are these "minor" materials a source of irritation and biocompatibility problems?

Does the material change its characteristics (physical and chemical) when sterilized? Do different types of sterilization have different effects? Are there long-term changes to the material because of the sterilization process? The choice of the sterilization method can have a profound effect on the safety and performance of a material or a device. If you use EtO sterilization on a material that is a significant barrier to gas, you may have a sterile product in the package, but if the ethylene oxide is trapped within the material you may have a potential toxicity problem.* Is there a difference† between electron-beam sterilization and gamma ray irradiation? Well, except for a few quantum mechanics, not a whole lot of scientific differences exist for the practicality of sterilization. However, some materials respond differently to the dose rate at which they are irradiated. Could this cause a potential problem? For most commonly used materials in medical devices the answer is *probably* not. But it's not true for all materials and should be considered. Polymers cross-link, degrade, or do nothing in the presence of radiation.‡ People often consider cross-linking as "good" and degradation as "bad." In fact, neither is either. If cross-linking results in a material that is now more brittle than is appropriate for a medical device, is that good? Still degradation is a problem and it doesn't always occur immediately. It wasn't that long ago when polypropylene syringes were sterilized by irradiation and were found to crack some months later.

Are there interactions of the materials with drugs that the patient may take? Have you ever seen a medical-grade adhesive that was working really well on a particular person for years and then one day stopped sticking? After an exhaustive study the only thing that seemed to have changed was that the person was receiving a new prescription drug. Was this a coincidence or a drug interaction? It was hard to tell, because there just wasn't sufficient information. An enormous amount of information is available today on drug interactions. Drugs are materials like anything else. Could they interact with your device or material?

Does anything in the literature suggest that the material or a closely related material has biocompatibility problems or

---

* This may be in addition to better-known packaging material problems with EtO.

† This is, of course, neglecting such mundane things as cost and product shape, etc.

‡ Actually, they do a little of everything.

is toxic? There are databases that contain a wealth of information on the toxicity and biocompatibility issues associated with different materials. The suppliers of the commercial products that you use can get you useful information from the very beginning. Some times it's even as simple as reading the material safety data sheet (MSDS) that came with the sample you requested. Sometimes you need a chemist to tell you the risk associated with your material based on its similarity to something else.

Many more questions need to be answered before a material could be considered safe and effective for use as a medical device itself or as a component of such a device. The fundamental question revolves around whether the device or material is sufficiently biocompatible for its intended application.

BIOCOMPATIBILITY

Biocompatibility is generally determined by tests using toxicological principles that provide information on the potential toxicity of materials in a clinical application. Many classical toxicological tests, however, were developed for a pure chemical agent and are not applicable to biocompatibility testing of materials and devices.

A biomaterial is usually a complex entity, and the material toxicity is affected by both physical and chemical properties. Toxicity from a biomaterial or polymer formulation often comes from components that migrate to the surface and are extracted from the material. The chemical composition of the material is often not known. Sometimes toxicological information on the material and its chemical composition is not available, and the possible interactions among the components in any given biological test system are often not known.

Biocompatibility cannot be defined by a single test. It is necessary to test as many biocompatibility parameters as possible. It is also important to test as many samples of the material as possible. Suitable positive and negative controls should be used and produce a standard response in repeated tests. The use of an exaggerated challenge, such as using higher dose ranges and longer contact durations or multiple insults that are many times more severe than the actual use condition, is important. Adopting an acceptable exposure level that is multiple factors below the lowest toxic level has also been a general practice.

Most of the biocompatibility tests to establish acute toxicity are short-term tests. Data from these short-term tests should not be overextended to cover the areas where no test results are available. Biocompatibility testing should be designed to assess the potential adverse effects under actual use conditions or specific conditions close to the actual use conditions. The physical and biological data obtained from biocompatibility tests should be correlated to the device and its use. Accuracy and reproducibility of these tests depend on the method and equipment used and often on the investigator's skill and experience.

You must consider several toxicological principles before planning biocompatibility testing. Biocompatibility depends on the tissue that contacts the device. For example, the requirements for a blood-contacting device would be different from those applicable to an external urinary catheter. The degree of biocompatibility assurance also depends on the involvement and the duration of contact with the human body.

Some materials, such as those used in orthopedic implants, are meant to last for a long period in the patient. In this case a biocompatibility test needs to show that the implant does not adversely affect the body during the long period of use. The possibility of biodegradation of the material or device should not be ignored. Biodegradation by the body can change an implant's safety and effectiveness. The materials leached from plastic used during a hemodialysis procedure may be very low, but the patient who is dialyzed three times a week may be exposed to a total of several grams during his or her lifetime. Therefore, cumulative effects should also be assessed when appropriate.

Two materials having the same chemical composition but different physical characteristics—for example, particle size—may *not* induce the same biological response. Also, past biological experience with seemingly identical materials is not necessarily indicative of biocompatibility in a new application. Toxicity may come from leachable components of the material due to differences in formulation and manufacturing procedures.

The empirical correlation between biocompatibility testing results and actual toxic findings in humans and the extrapolation of the quantitative results from short-term *in-vitro* tests to quantitative toxicity at the time of use are controversial. These need careful and scientifically sound interpretation and adjustment.

The challenge of biocompatibility testing is to use the knowledge to reduce the degree of unknowns and to help make the logical decisions. The hazard presented by a substance, with its inherent toxic potential, can only be truly known when the material is actually exposed to a patient. Therefore, risk is a function of toxic hazard and exposure. The safety of any materials that may migrate from a device or are contained in the device or on its surface can be evaluated by determining the total amount of potentially harmful substance, estimating the amount reaching the patient tissues, assessing the risk of exposure, and performing a risk-versus-benefit analysis. When the potential harm from the use of the biomaterial is identified from the biocompatibility tests, this potential must be compared against the availability of an alternate material.

REGULATORY ASPECTS OF BIOCOMPATIBILITY

Basic biocompatibility guidance is found in the document *Tripartite Biocompatibility for Medical Devices*, which provides a suitable framework to test for biocompatibility. This document is from the Toxicology Subgroup of the Tripartite Subcommittee on Medical Devices of Canada, the United Kingdom, and the United States. The Tripartite guidance recommends the application of fundamental principles to determine the appropriateness of biocompatibility testing.

To evaluate the safety of medical devices, the guidance categorizes medical devices based on the type of body contact. The biological tests required depend on the body contact and contact duration. See Table 1, which lists the biological tests that might be applied for evaluating the safety of medical devices made of polymers. It does not imply that all tests listed under each category are necessary. The tests can be modified to accommodate devices made of metals, ceramics, or biological materials.

Medical device manufacturers need to be careful about using *generally recognized as safe* (GRAS) substances. GRAS

Table 1 Biological Tests—Biomaterials

Level I		
Acute	Screening tests	Cytotoxicity
		USP biological tests
		Hemolysis
	Other tests	Irritation
		Sensitization
		Implantation
		Hemocompatibility
		Mutagenicity
		Reproductive
		Pyrogenicity
Subchronic & chronic		Irritation
		Sensitization
		Implantation
		Hemocompatibility
		Reproductive & developmental
Level II	Chronic	Implantation
		Reproductive & developmental
		Carcinogenesis
		Additional tests based on Level I, e.g., pharmacokinetics
Level III	Clinical studies	

substances can be found in 21 CFR Part 182; they are applicable to food but are not directly applicable to medical devices. Any material or substance in the GRAS list cannot automatically be assumed as safe and effective for medical devices.

Biocompatibility Testing Programs

Manufacturers must devise a biocompatibility test program that involves some or all of the following activities:

- Gather information on the material and the finished device.
- Complete a physio-chemical characterization of the material.
- Identify rapid, sensitive, cost-effective screening tests.
- Monitor incoming raw materials, the final product, and the manufacturing process.
- Define the product release tests and the pass/fail criteria.

In addition, the manufacturer should select reliable, state-of-the-art bioassays to demonstrate safety for the intended use of the device.

Regulatory issues are equally as complex as the scientific considerations. Some regulatory issues are

- Anticipated human exposure to the device
- Biological resistance to chemical insult
- Testing variables
- Species differences
- Relevance of the test to the device and its use
- Substantiating the accuracy and predictive values of the test
- Proper interpretation
- The use of no observed biological responses (negative results) to chemical insult(s) to predict biocompatibility

Undesirable extremes should be avoided during the design of biocompatibility testing programs. It is important not to attempt to demonstrate biocompatibility by a single test, and a biocompatibility program should be based on the intended use of the device. The large number of tests and test samples is as important as the accuracy, specificity, significance, and economy of the testing. Medical devices vary widely in their types, uses, functions, exposures, and contact ions. Therefore, one test system cannot accommodate all applications. Manufacturers *do not* have to repeat extensive biocompatibility testing programs simply to fill the files of evidence of safety *if the device is constructed of well-known, previously well-tested materials, or only uses materials with a long, safe history for the same intended use.*

Some tests may be inappropriate or unnecessary for the intended use of the device. For example, pyrogenicity tests are appropriate for intravenous catheters but not for topical devices that contact only intact external surfaces. Figure 4 lists suggested biocompatibility tests.

PHASES OF BIOCOMPATIBILITY TESTING

Good biocompatibility testing programs for medical devices should follow three levels of testing. See Table 1.

- Level I tests include information on the physical and chemical characterization of the materials and screening toxicological tests. Level I tests are generally not difficult to perform, require readily available equipment, and are considered a minimal characterization of biomaterials. These tests have broad application and low resolution and are recommended for screening during the early stages of development and continued monitoring of new lots of materials.
- Level II tests involve acute toxicity tests and some subchronic and chronic tests if needed. Level II testing

Device categories			Biological effect											
Body contact		Contact duration	Initial evaluation tests								Supplementary tests			
		A = limited, less than 24 hours; B = prolonged, 24 hours to 30 days; C = permanent, greater than 30 days	Cytotoxicity	Sensitization	Irritation/intracutaneous reactivity	Systemic toxicity (acute)	Subchronic toxicity	Genotoxicity	Implantation	Hemocompatibility	Chronic Toxicity	Carcinogenicity	Reproductive/developmental (3)	Biodegradation (3)
Surface devices	Skin	A	X	X	X									
		B	X	X	X									
		C	X	X	X									
	Mucosal membrane	A	X	X	X									
		B	X	X	X	O	O		O					
		C	X	X	X	O	X	X	O		O			
	Breached/compromised surface	A	X	X	X	O								
		B	X	X	X	O	O		O					
		C	X	X	X	O	X	X	O		O			
External communicating devices	Indirect blood path	A	X	X	X	X				X				
		B	X	X	X	X	O			X				
		C	X	X	O	X	X	X	O	X	X	X		
	Tissue/bone communicating (2)	A	X	X	X	O								
		B	X	X	O	O	O	X	X					
		C	X	X	O	O	O	X	X		O	X		
	Circulating blood	A	X	X	X	X		O (2)		X				
		B	X	X	X	X	O	X	O	X				
		C	X	X	X	X	X	X	O	X	X	X		
Implant devices	Tissue/bone	A	X	X	X	O								
		B	X	X	O	O	O	X	X					
		C	X	X	O	O	O	X	X		X	X		
	Blood	A	X	X	X	X			X	X				
		B	X	X	X	X	O	X	X	X				
		C	X	X	X	X	X	X	X	X	X	X		

Notes: *X= ISO test*
O= Additional tests that may be applicable
(1) Includes tissue fluids and subcutaneous spaces
(2) For all devices used in extracorporeal circuits
(3) Depends on device and component materials

Figure 4 Suggested biocompatibility testing.

is basically an extension of Level I and involves a variety of *in-vitro* and *in-vivo* testing of devices that require additional testing based on the Level I screening tests. This includes extensive preclinical tests such as pharmacokinetic studies and lifetime bioassays or special testing due to complexity and/or intended use of the device.

- Level III testing involves clinical studies. Manufacturers should determine whether or not to proceed to Level II or Level III testing depending on the results of Level I tests.

Screening Tests

Screening tests allow rapid and relatively inexpensive rejection of incompatible materials at an early stage and can be used as a monitoring device of the manufacturing process. The cytotoxicity tests, intracutaneous and/or skin irritation tests, and hemolysis tests are good candidates for screening. In addition, many cell or tissue culture systems can be custom-tailored to biomaterials. Unless clearly contraindicated, both direct-contact tests and tests with extract with polar and nonpolar extraction media should be considered.

Some manufacturers overestimate the importance of screening tests alone as a proof of biocompatibility. These screening tests are not intended to demonstrate that the material is biocompatible, but to reject grossly incompatible materials.

Acute Toxicity Tests

Biomaterial testing strategy has been broadly established as acute, subchronic, and chronic.

- *Acute* toxicity is generally a toxic effect resulting from short-term exposure, usually less than 30 days, to a chemical substance. Biological tests for acute toxicity include estimates of irritation, sensitization potential,

cytotoxicity, hematologic profile, and evaluation of the local toxic effect on living tissue by surgical implantation.
- *Subchronic* toxicity is generally a toxic effect resulting either from prolonged exposure up to 90 days or from multiple exposures.
- *Chronic* toxicity is generally a toxic effect from continuous and prolonged exposure.

The most common cause of acute toxicity of a biomaterial is the presence of biologically active leachable substances, and the acute toxic responses are closely related to the kind and quantity of leachable substances in or on the materials or devices. Although the absence of leachable substances is desired, extraction procedures will yield detectable quantities of chemical substances. It is important to assess the potential toxic effect of the material and to keep in mind the potential toxic effect of apparently minor or undetected substances.

Toxicity testing should be used in conjunction with chemical and physical analysis to prevent costly development of unsatisfactory materials. The acute toxic response of materials comes from the presence and leachability of toxic substances. Therefore, the detection of leachable substances should be the principal focus of the test systems. Tests can be performed directly on the material, on the device, or on the extracts.

If a leachable substance is contained and cannot migrate to the surface at the time of the testing, the results will appear to be satisfactory for a short test. The substance will be exposed and becomes leachable when the polymer degrades after a longer period of time. Devices intended for longer duration must be tested for longer periods according to subchronic or chronic test methods.

Acute toxicity does not necessarily predict potential harmful effects from longer exposures, multiple exposures, bioaccumulation, biodegradation, delayed responses, carcinogenicity, and reproductive toxicity. The duration of subchronic or chronic studies should be appropriate to the expected duration of use.

If the FDA requires Level II subchronic or chronic tests, manufacturers should consult the CDRH's Office of Device Evaluation before running the test programs.

TESTS TO DEMONSTRATE BIOCOMPATIBILITY

Cytotoxicity and Cell Cultures

Cell culture tests including cytotoxicity are a good predictor of biocompatibility when used together with other appropriate tests. Several highly specialized cell culture methods are available to monitor the biocompatibility of the raw materials used in the manufacturing of the device or auditing of the manufacturing process. Cell or tissue culture testing offers several advantages:

- It is simple, rather inexpensive, and easy to perform.
- It allows testing of a biomaterial on human tissue.
- It is sensitive to toxic material.
- It is easy to manipulate and allows more than one end-point investigation.
- It can be used to construct a dose-response curve.
- It can give quick and quantitative results and allows direct access or direct observation or measurement.

Although cell or tissue cultures offer many advantages, their use is limited to screening the biomaterials. Therefore, cytotoxicity results should be used for biocompatibility only in conjunction with other tests.

Many tissue culture methods are available for testing of biomaterials. These are divided into two major groups: One tests the toxicity of a soluble extract of the material, and the other tests the toxicity by the direct contact of cells with the material or components of the device.

Examples of cytotoxicity test methods using extracts include

- *Fluid medium tissue culture* that evaluates the cellular damage caused by the test extract on a confluent monolayer culture. The test extract is incorporated into the culture medium. The toxic effect on the monolayer, such as cell lysis and microscopic observation of cell morphology changes, is usually checked after 24 and 48 hours. Cell lysis can be scored by direct microscopic observation or with the use of radiolabels or blue-dye uptake.
- The *inhibition of cell growth* is a more informative test requiring more time and skill. Distilled water extract is incorporated into the tissue culture medium and inoculated with the cells in the tissue culture tubes. After 72 hours the extent of cell growth is determined by total protein assay on the cells removed from the individual tubes.
- The *cloning efficiency assay* is even more informative, sensitive, and quantitative and requires even more skill. The cloning efficiency assay's procedure and endpoint is similar but is more accurate, sensitive, and direct than the cell growth inhibition or fluid medium method. The cloning efficiency assay normally uses a Chinese hamster ovary cell line and a single-cell cloning technique to estimate the toxic insult-induced reduction in cloning efficiency. The cytotoxic effect of the extract is determined by measuring the ability of the treated cells to form colonies during seven subsequent days of incubation. The cloning efficiency of the treated cultures is compared to that of the control. The agar overlay method can be used to evaluate the toxicity of the extracts, but it is primarily used for the direct-contact cytotoxicity tests of the solid test sample.

Several tests are available to test cytotoxicity by direct contact. These include

1. ASTM F 813 Practice for Direct Contact Cell Culture Evaluation of Materials for Medical Devices
2. ASTM F 1027 Standard Practice for Assessment of Tissue and Cell Compatibility on Prosthetic Materials and Devices
3. NIH Publication No. 85-2185 Guidelines for Blood–Material Interactions
4. HIMA Report Guidelines for the Preclinical Safety Evaluation of Materials Used in Medical Devices
5. Others including many device specific toxicity guidance documents on toxicity testing

In addition, the agar overlay tissue culture method and fluid medium tissue culture method can be used for direct-contact cytotoxicity testing. In the fluid medium method the test material or device is placed directly on the growing monolayer cell surface. In the agar overlay method the solid test sample is placed on or in the agar layer containing vital stain such as neutral red over the growing monolayer of cells. The response is evaluated grossly and microscopically and graded according to the zone index, the size of the cytopathic area, the lysis index, and percent of cell. (See Table 2) Proper cytotoxicity testing must include at least one test with extract and one direct-contact test.

In addition, differentiated cells are used to evaluate the effects materials may have on specific tissues. Differentiated cells are generally nonfibroblastic cells that are different from transformed and fibroblastic cell lines such as L-cells used in ASTM cytotoxicity test methods. Differentiated cells have organ-specific or tissue-specific functions and have specific biological endpoints or measurable characteristics. Liver cells, which are differentiated cells, have all or some liver functions.

Table 2 Cell Lysis Zone Index

Lysis index	Extent of cell lysis
0	None observable
1	Less than 20%
2	Less than 40%
3	Less than 60%
4	Greater than 60%
Zone Index	**Description of zone**
0	No detectable zone
1	Limited to area under sample
2	Less than 0.5 cm from sample
3	Less than 1.0 cm from sample
4	Greater than 1.0 cm

Note: A score other than 0 should be studied further. A score greater than 2 should be evaluated for potential harm.

Most cells in culture are fibroblasts. Primary cells that are taken directly from an animal are difficult to establish in culture and become fibroblasts, losing the normal functions of growing differentiated cells. Numerous conditions have to be optimized for obtaining good growth in differentiated cells. Most cultured cells have a fibroblastic appearance, although they may not be fibroblasts. The fibroblasts in culture can take over cultures because they readily grow on plastic surfaces. The recent success in growing differentiated cells was partially due to technique that have been developed to remove and limit the growth of fibroblasts to allow other cells to grow. The properties of the cell cultures usually depend on the cultivation conditions, and normal cells grow in culture only for a limited number of generations.

The test in differentiated cells is important for at least two reasons. First, the tissue-type specific features of differentiated cells may modulate the effects of chemicals on the fundamental properties of cells. Second, it is important to determine the effects of chemicals on specific cell function responses.

Many companies consider that the *in-vitro* cytotoxicity test correlates well with other screening acute toxicity tests such as USP VI, but is more sensitive. The FDA considers that cytotoxicity tests are good replacements for the systemic test in mice, which the FDA no longer supports. All materials, in general, should be subjected to a cytotoxicity test, which is the *in-vitro* test intended to predict possible toxicity. The failure of a device or material to pass an *in-vitro* tissue culture test needs thorough review.

USP Biological Tests

Several USP biological reactivity tests are designed to test the suitability of materials intended for use in fabricating containers or accessories for parenteral preparations test the suitability of polymers for medical use in implants.

- The systemic injection test and intracutaneous test are designed to determine the biological response of animals to plastics by single-dose injection of specific extracts prepared from a sample.
- The implantation test is designed to evaluate the reaction of living tissue to the plastic by the implantation of the sample into animal tissue. The use of the systemic injection test in mice is no longer recommended by the FDA's CDRH.
- The intracutaneous test is designed to score the inflammatory reaction that may occur after the test extract has been injected into the rabbit's skin. The intramuscular implantation in rabbits macroscopically examines the area of the tissue surrounding the center portion of each implant strip.

Many manufacturers use the USP Class VI test for demonstrating biocompatibility to the FDA. Class VI requires extracts using sodium chloride, alcohol in sodium chloride, polyethylene glycol, and vegetable oil. Class IV requires one less extraction, which is polyethylene glycol. Even though the

Class VI is a well-recognized predictor of biocompatibility, it may have little relevance to the biocompatibility evaluation of the intended use of the device. Other tests for biocompatibility can be used to resolve specific questions regarding intended use.

Irritation Tests

Intracutaneous Tests

The intracutaneous irritation Test is a sensitive acute toxicity-screening test and is generally accepted for detecting potential local irritation by extracts from a biomaterial. Extracts of material obtained with nonirritating polar and nonpolar extraction media are suitable, and sterile extracts are desirable. Rabbits are the most commonly used animals. A more detailed description can be found in *Biological Reactivity Tests, In Vivo, Intracutaneous Test*, and ASTM F749 *Standard Practice for Evaluating Material Extracts by Intracutaneous Injection in the Rabbit*. The irritation results are evaluated on a scale of 0 to 4, from "no erythema" (0) to "severe" (4). A similar scale is used for edema. The result is the average value obtained from five animals. Any score greater than 2 should be evaluated for potential harm. The methods of testing primary (skin) irritant substances can be found in the Code of Federal Regulations: 16 CFR 1500.40, 1500.41, and 1500.42.

Skin irritation testing is performed to demonstrate the potential toxicity of the device, that is, initiating or aggravating damage through its contact with the skin. Primary skin irritation is usually done according to the regulations of the Consumer Product Safety Commission, Title 16, Chapter II, Part 1500. The purpose of the test is to determine the dermal irritation potential of the article to the intact and abraded skin of the rabbit.

Dermal Sensitization Study (Animal Study)

Dermal sensitization is performed to demonstrate the potential of the device for eliciting an immunological response through its contact with the skin. This reaction is due primarily to substances that could leach out of a material. Guinea pigs are used because they have been shown to be the best animal model for human allergic contact dermatitis.*

Modified Draize Test (Human Study)

John Draize of the FDA developed the *Draize test*. The test uses albino rabbits to test cosmetics, toiletries, pesticides, drugs, and other products. The test was designed to assess the eye irritancy of chemicals and mixtures of chemicals. The test results are scored according to Title 16, Chapter II, Parts 1500.41 and 1500.3(c)(4).

Ocular Irritation tests

The requirements for the USP Eye Irritation Test and Three Week Ocular Irritation Test in Rabbits can be found in the FDA'S Guidance Document for Class III Contact Lenses. This document prepared by the Office of Device Evaluation can be obtained through the Division of Small Manufacturers Assistance (DSMA).

Sensitization Tests

Sensitization tests are used to determine adverse effects mediated by immunological mechanisms from material after repeated or prolonged exposure. Sensitization is a delayed hypersensitivity reaction and is manifested in a variety of clinical complications. Hypersensitivity is the condition of a primed individual who tends to give an exaggerated immunological response on further exposure to the relevant antigen. When an individual has been immunologically primed or sensitized, further contact with the antigen can not only lead to secondary boosting of the immune response but can also cause

---

* ASTM Standard F-720 Standard Practice for Testing Guinea Pig Contact Allergens, Guinea Pig Maximization Test.

tissue-damaging reactions. There is no test to reliably and accurately predict the sensitization potential of biomaterials. However, the ASTM Standard Practice for Testing Guinea Pigs for Contact Allergens; Guinea Pig Maximization Test (ASTM F720) is widely used to determine the potential for a substance or material extract to elicit contact dermal allergenicity. Immediate allergy skin testing (IAST) is a very useful and sensitive hypersensitivity test. Two such *in-vitro* tests, the lymphocyte transformation test and inhibition of macrophage migration, have been used as an alternative to the skin patch testing.

Hemocompatibility Tests

The term "hemocompatibility" should be used only in a defined context. Few materials have consistently shown good hemocompatibility in both arterial and venous blood-flow environments. Results obtained from laboratory animals may not apply to man, and results from one test system cannot be correlated to those obtained from a different test system. Any hemocompatibility statement should be linked to the intended use and conditions for which the statement is valid.

The blood–material interaction can range from minimal protein adsorption to activation of coagulation, complement, and destruction of cells. Complicated mechanisms exist in the cardiovascular system that interacts with medical devices. Devices vary enormously in type, function, and duration of blood contact. Therefore, a multidisciplinary approach to hemocompatibility testing is important. This includes *in-vitro* static and dynamic tests, acute extracorporeal tests, tests of cardiovascular devices in animals, and clinical studies. This section will be limited to static *in-vitro* tests. For other, more specialized tests, manufacturers should consult with hemocompatibility experts or the Office of Device Evaluation (ODE).

Hemolysis Tests

Hemolysis tests evaluate the acute *in-vitro* hemolytic properties of materials, especially those led for use in contact with blood. The concentration of substances that produce hemolysis is generally higher than that needed to produce a cytotoxic effect. The results of hemolysis testing can be correlated with acute *in-vivo* toxicity tests. A hemolysis test is rapid, requires simple equipment and easily interpretable quantitative results, and can be performed in the presence of the material of the extract. The results are compared to the controls and expressed as percent hemolysis. The ASTM F756 Standard Practice for Assessment of Hemolytic Properties of Materials can be used to measure hemolytic potential.

Erythrocyte Stability

The erythrocyte stability test provides a sensitive measure of the interaction of leachable substances with the plasma membrane of erythrocytes and is reflected as changes in the osmotic fragility of the erythrocytes. This test can detect leachables at concentrations slightly below the levels of many cytotoxicity systems.

Protein Adsorption

The adsorption of plasma protein is generally the first event that occurs when blood contacts a foreign surface. This protein layer has a great influence on the thrombogenicity of a material. One of the more commonly used techniques is the radio labeling of protein with ^{125}I. This technique provides a direct measurement of the amount of protein adsorbed on a surface.

Implantation Tests

Two examples of implantation tests are the Standard Practice for Short-Term Screening Implant Material (ASTM F763) and Standard Practice for Assessment of Compatibility Biomaterials (Nonporous) for Surgical Implants with Respect to Effect of Materials on Muscle and Bone (ASTM F981).

Mutagenicity Tests

Genetic and cell culture techniques are available to test mutagenic properties to demonstrate the presence or lack of ability of the test material to cause mutation or chromosomal damage or cancer. The material intended for intimate contact and long exposure should not have any mutagenic properties. The presence of nonpolymerized materials and traces of monomers, oligomers, additives, or biodegradation products can cause mutations.

Mutation can be either a point mutation or a chromosomal rearrangement caused by DNA damage. Therefore, the material's ability to cause point mutation, chromosomal change, or evidence of DNA damage should be tested. Correlations exist between mutagenic and carcinogenic properties. Most, if not all, carcinogens are mutagens, but not all mutagens are human carcinogens.

- The Ames salmonella/microsome test is a principal sensitive mutagen-screening test. Compounds are tested on the mutants of *Salmonella typhimuriun* for reversion from a histidine requirement back to prototrophy. A positive result is seen by the growth of revertant bacteria. A microsomal activation system should be included in this assay. The use of all five bacterial test strains is generally required. Two nonbacterial mutagenicity tests are generally required to support the lack of mutagenic or carcinogenic potential.

Pyrogenicity Tests

Pyrogenicity testing is generally required if

- The label claims that the device is pyrogen-free.
- The device comes in contact with blood or spinal fluid.
- The device is an intraocular lens.

Reproductive and Developmental Toxicity

Irreversible toxic effects are associated with adverse reactions of the reproductive system and in the offspring. Reproductive anomalies range from sterility to problems in the production of the mother's milk. The adverse influence may occur at any time within the reproductive cycle of the organism. Toxic effects to the offspring range from mortality to morbidity as subtle as decreased body weight at birth. Pronounced reproductive anomalies are teratic or morphological defects observed in offspring at birth. Teratology has expanded to include not only morphological alterations but also biochemical, immunological, and behavioral deficits.

Carcinogenesis Bioassays

The carcinogenesis bioassays observe the test animal over a major portion of its life span for the development of neoplastic lesions. Because of the long latent period required for induction and manifestation of tumors, it is necessary to expose the test animals when young and continue for duration of the experiment. The organs and tissues of both treated and control animals should be examined for morphological changes. The absence of a carcinogenic effect cannot be assured unless all organ systems have been examined with high accuracy in all animals, and all grossly visible suspect lesions examined microscopically. More comprehensive carcinogenesis protocols can be found in the FDA's Toxicological Principles for the Safety Assessment of Direct Food Additives and Color Additives Used in Food.

9

Process Validation

IT'S NO GOOD IF YOU CAN'T MAKE IT

Strictly speaking, process validation is not part of design controls. But the best product design in the world is useless if it can't be made in a consistent and efficient way and at an appropriate cost. At least it's not part of Subpart C on design controls although design validation must occur on initial production units or their equivalent. So it would make little sense to get that far along in the developmental process without having developed and validated the process by which the product is going to be made. In fact, the very next step after design validation in formal design control is design transfer, which involves getting everything out of development and moving it into manufacturing. The time to start worrying about how the product will ultimately be made is Day 2 of the development program; the day after the product is designated as a probable commercial product, not the day you start the design validation run.

Back at the beginning of the book, we mention in passing that very few people would go to a bagel store to buy an emerald ring. Well, there are a few jewelers that you probably wouldn't go to either. In order to make a perfect emerald ring, you need more than a good natural emerald and some gold. You need a manufacturing process. Natural emeralds are hard to find, and once you've found one that is valuable, you don't want someone who's cutting emeralds for the first time working on your particular stone. You want to have a system that will cut the emerald correctly the first time it is struck. You also want it polished and set correctly. Therefore, you wouldn't turn the gem over to someone who has never cut and polished a natural emerald before. Neither should you attempt to manufacture a medical device without first knowing how you intend to make it *and* having the assurance that the process will produce the product according to the specifications set during the design control process.

THE FDA AND PROCESS VALIDATION

The FDA does talk about process validation in 21 CFR 820, not in Subpart C for Design Controls, but in Subpart G, Production and Process Controls. In Section 820.75 it says

> (a) Where the results of a process cannot fully be verified by subsequent inspection and test, the process shall be validated with a high degree of assurance and approved according to established procedures. The validation activities and results, including the date and signature of the individual(s) approving the validation and where appropriate the major equipment validated, shall be documented.

(b) Each manufacturer shall establish and maintain procedures for monitoring and control of process parameters for validated processes to ensure that specification requirements continue to be met.
(1) Each manufacturer shall ensure that validated processes are performed by qualified individuals.
(2) For validated processes, the monitoring and the control methods and data, the date performed, and, where appropriate, the individual(s) performing the process or the major equipment used shall be documented.

(c) When changes or process deviations occur, the manufacturer shall review and evaluate the process and perform revalidation where appropriate. These activities shall be documented.

A model operating procedure for process control is shown in Appendix G.

WHAT DO YOU CALL A GROUP OF PROCESSES?

If you can have a litter of puppies or a pride of lions, what do you call a group of processes strung together to make a medical device? Manufacturing, of course! In the manufacturing of many medical devices, several different operations are tied together to make the device. Let's look in Figure 1 at the manufacturing process for making a colostomy pouch.

Although oversimplified, Figure 1 shows the need for validation of this manufacturing process, or at least some of the five subprocesses that are part of this manufacturing setup. We have identified five separate processes necessary for the manufacture of a relatively simple medical device. This device is actually a class I product, so it is not necessary to establish a design control program for it in the first place. But as we said before there are many reasons, including quality and the company's bottom line, for doing so.

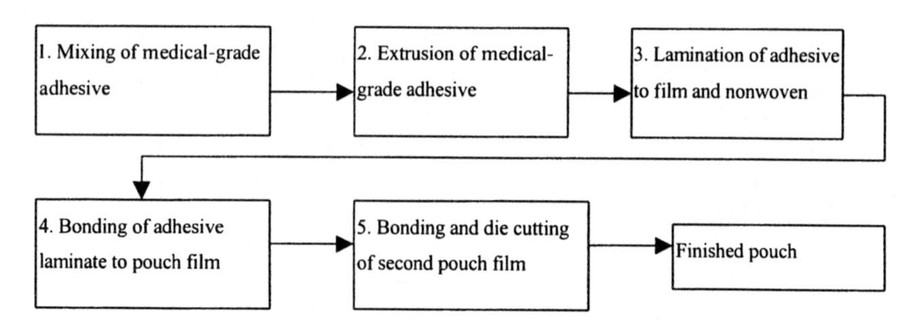

Figure 1 Typical manufacturing process for a one-piece colostomy pouch.

The first question we need to ask is which, if any, of these processes should be validated? The FDA says, "Where the results of a process cannot fully be verified by subsequent inspection and test, the process shall be validated."

The first step of the overall manufacturing process is the mixing of the medical-grade adhesive that serves as the means for holding the pouch on the patient and protecting the patient's skin. Typically such an adhesive formulation might contain up to a dozen separate ingredients.* These ingredients are mixed together in separate batches according to a procedure that specifies the order of addition, the temperature at critical points in the mixing, and the length of time the mixing is allowed to run for each addition of raw materials or group of raw materials. Change any of those things beyond a certain range and the resultant adhesive may have different properties.

Assume that the development work has led to an adhesive with an ideal set of properties for the application and that this was verified through standard adhesive testing such as

* If the adhesive is not an acrylic or a urethane but is the typical "hydrocolloid" adhesive used in many ostomy pouches.

tack, shear, and peel adhesion.* Assume further that this was validated by skin adhesion tests on volunteer subjects and with an actual clinical use test of the device. How do you know whether each batch of material made in production is the same as the adhesive made and tested during the development of the product? Can you test (verify) that each batch is the same as the one before and after and that each of these is what was developed and verified previously? The answer is "yes," maybe. An appropriate sample of each batch can be taken when the mix is completed and subject to a battery of adhesion tests in order to verify that they meet the specifications that were developed. If you have a good correlation between these *in-vitro* tests and *in-vivo* results, you have verification, thus validating that this subprocess is not necessary. There are, however, several potential problems. First, the correlation between adhesion in the lab and adhesion to people probably isn't as good as you think. The same person using the same adhesive batch may have different results from day to day. Diet, drugs, exercise, ambient temperature, and humidity change things. Stainless steel, the most often used test substrate, does not undergo these changes. Having human subjects hanging around to act as test substrates doesn't seem quite practical either. Second, the batch mixing process is slow compared to the other processes that come after it. It may not be practical to have everyone wait for the slowest Boy Scout marching† along in the line before proceeding with the rest of the process. So maybe a validated mixing process is a benefit.

Of course, there is at least one way to verify that the batch is consistent with the product specifications. During the development a correlation between both the *in-vivo* and *in-vitro* ad-

---

* Let's assume the testing was done at 40°C to simulate body temperature and we weren't misled by results observed at room temperature.

† If you want to know where the Boy Scout came from and about optimizing production, read *The Goal* by Goldratt and Cox, North River Press, 1984.

hesion results could have been made with some property intrinsic to the material. If the right instrumentation is available, this method could be used to verify that each batch of medical-grade adhesive made according to the established procedure and containing the right amounts of all the required materials meets the product specifications.*

All in all, it may be a good idea to validate this batch subprocess. It would allow a smoother flow into the rest of the manufacturing steps for a subprocess that is already time-consuming. Here's what can be done:

1. For each of the ingredients one needs to determine the added range beyond which the formula no longer achieves the specified properties using a constant mix procedure. When this allowable variation for each ingredient is known, the mix process itself can be validated.

2. Using a designed experiment,† the process parameters (time, order of ingredient addition, temperature) should be evaluated at several points above, below, and at the optimum conditions set during the development. This set of conditions encompassing upper and lower processing limits and circumstances, including those within standard operating procedures, pose the greatest chance of process or product failure when compared to "ideal" conditions. Remember that such conditions do not necessarily induce product or process failure.

3. Each batch should then be carefully tested according to standard test methods and the results statistically evaluated to determine the parameters of the process. A multiple regression analysis of the results may even illuminate which parameter is more critical than the others.

Now what about the extrusion? Validate or rely on verification. Here the answer depends primarily on what your ex-

---

* If you don't know how to do this, we're not telling you. We're consultants, remember? All you have to do is hire us to find out.

† A good example of the value of DOE in process validation can be seen in M.J. Anderson and P.J. Anderson, Design of experiments for process validation, *Medical Device & Diagnostic Industry*, January 1999, pp. 193–199.

truder has in terms of inline inspection instrumentation or how much you would be willing to spend to equip the unit to make the necessary measurements while the extruder is running. Many of the physical properties of the exudate such as width and thickness can be quickly and easily made offline using appropriate sampling techniques during a run. At the same time inline measurement gauges are readily available and continuously monitor thickness and keep necessary documentation. Remember that the use of such equipment will require validation of that component. But what about the effects of the extrusion temperature profile, the residence time in the barrel (screw speed), and the backpressure? Assuming the development work was done correctly, these parameters were set and are all interrelated. So the product of the extrusion could be easily handled with simple testing. The exception is the extrusion of a heat-sensitive material that significantly changes properties depending on its heat history. In this case the extrusion subprocess should also be validated in a manner similar to that as outlined in the batch mixing subprocess.

The laminating process seems to be more easily handled through verification that the lamination has developed sufficient bond strength between the layers to prevent separation during anticipated use conditions. For large-scale, multishift operations a case could be made for validation of the process and control of the specified result by evaluating the nip roll pressures and temperatures as well as the line speed through the unit. One could then arrive at a set of conditions that would allow reasonable assurance that the specified lamination was accomplished as long as the parameters remained within the validated values.

The remaining die cutting and bonding* subprocesses are easily verifiable against product specifications using standard test methods, a proper sampling technique, and appropriate maintenance of the cutting dies. A strong case could be made

* These techniques include RF welding, heat sealing, or ultrasonic welding.

for the validation of any bonding machine such as an ultrasonic welder especially if this bonding occurs offline. If the bonding of the pouch outline weld was made through an RF weld, verification would be absolutely necessary whether or not the RF generator was validated, as RF welding in such an application is known to cause pinholes in the film due to arcing.

In general it should be remembered that

- All processes vary.
- Some processes vary more than others.
- Each variation has a cause, and many of these causes can be identified.
- To the extent that the causes can be identified and understood, they can be controlled.
- Only a few of the causes are significant; the greater the extent of control on these critical causes, the better control there is of the manufacturing process.
- The product design must be flexible enough to take up the remaining process variations.
- If it can't be manufactured efficiently with a high level of reproducible quality at a cost that will allow a profit, then you haven't got a product.

Once a process is validated, the need for inspection and testing is decreased dramatically and manufacturing can take advantage of statistical process control (SPC) methods to increase efficiency and throughput.

STATISTICAL PROCESS CONTROL

Processes and Process Variability

The concept of process variability, as outlined in the previous section, is the basis of statistical process control. As an example, suppose a marksman shoots 100 rounds at a target every day. He would not get the same number of shots at the center of the target during each daily session. Some days he would get 89 of 100, some days 73 of 100, some days 84 of 100, etc. All manufacturing processes have this kind of variation.

This process variation can be divided into two components. *Natural process variation,* or system variation, is the naturally occurring variation inherent in all processes. In the case of the shooter, this variation would vary around his long-term percentage of bulls-eye's hit. *Special cause variation* is caused by some problem or unusual occurrence in the system. In the case of our shooter, an eye infection would cause him to miss a larger than "normal" number of shots on that day.

Statistical process control is a method for graphically representing the process and determining when a process is "out of control." A process is out of control by this definition not because of its normal or inherent variation but because a special cause variation is present. Something unusual is occurring in the process. The process can then investigated to determine the base cause of this out-of-control condition. When the cause of the problem is determined, an action can be identified to correct it. The investigation and corrective action are a team process.

It is management's responsibility to reduce system variation as well as special cause variation. This is often accomplished through

- Process improvement techniques
- Investment in new technology
- Reengineering the process to have fewer steps and therefore less variation

Reduced variation makes the process more predictable, with process output closer to the specified value. This goal of minimal variation mandates working toward the goal of reduced process variation.

The process in Figure 2 is in apparent statistical control. All points lie within the upper control limit (UCL) and the lower control limit (LCL). This process is showing only normal

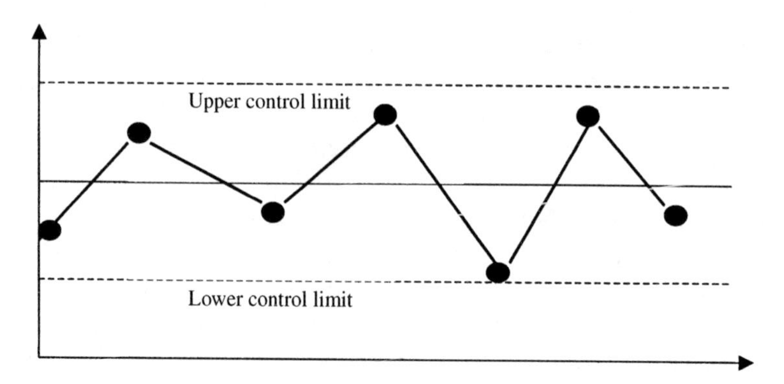

Figure 2 A process in statistical control.

system variation. The process charted in Figure 3 is out of statistical control. A single point can be found outside the control limits. This means that a special occurrence likely caused the variation above the upper control limit. There is small probability that this variation happened by chance, so when a point is found outside the control limits, it is very probable that a source of special cause variation occurred. This needs to be isolated and corrected. A single point outside the control limits is easily detectable as an out-of-control condition.

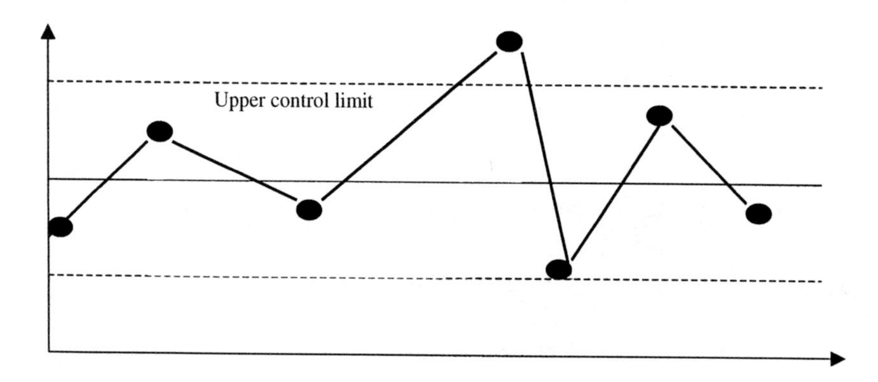

Figure 3 A process out of statistical control.

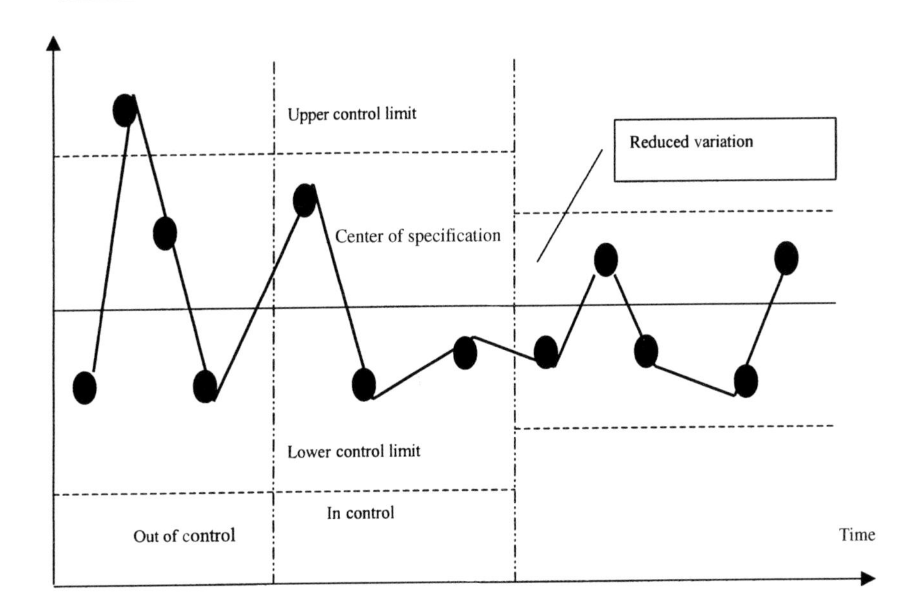

Figure 4 A process improvement cycle.

Figure 4 illustrates an SPC improvement cycle. The process begins out of specification (out of control), then, as causes of variation are found and corrective action is implemented, the process comes into statistical control. Through continuous process improvement, variation is reduced and a new specification representing a higher-quality product can be introduced. Eliminating special cause variation keeps the process in control; process improvement reduces the process variation and moves the control limits toward the center of the product specification.

Control Chart Zones

Control charts can be broken into three zones—A, B, and C—on each side of the process center specification. This is illustrated in Figure 5. Rules exist that are used to detect conditions in which the process is behaving in an out-of-control condition.

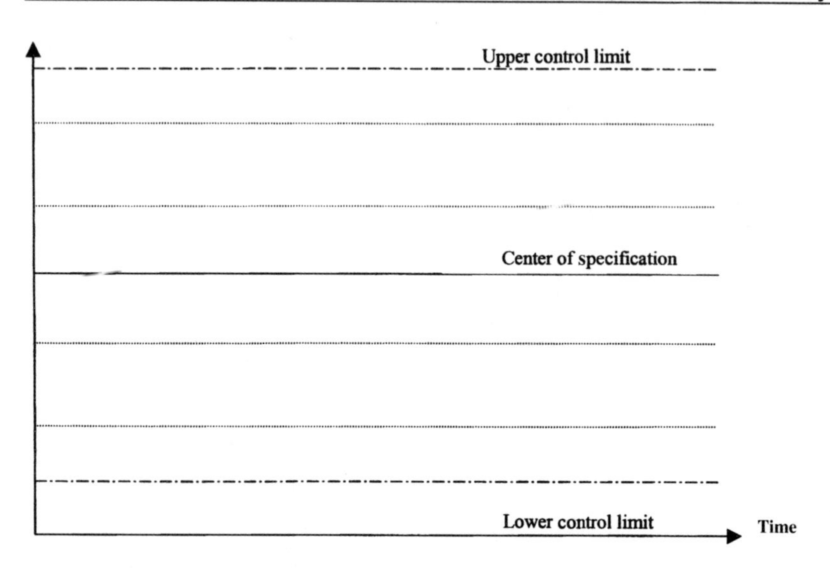

Figure 5 SPC control chart zones.

- The probability of having two out of three consecutive points either in or beyond zone A is an extremely unlikely occurrence when the process mean follows a normal distribution.
- The probability of having four out of five consecutive points either in or beyond zone B is also an extremely unlikely occurrence when the process mean follows the normal distribution.
- The probability of having eight or more consecutive points either above or below the centerline is also an extremely unlikely occurrence when the process follows the normal distribution.
- The probability of six or more consecutive points showing a continuous increase or decrease is also an extremely unlikely occurrence when the process follows the normal distribution.
- The probability of having 14 or more consecutive points oscillating back and forth is also an extremely

unlikely occurrence when the process follows the normal distribution.

- The probability of having eight or more consecutive points occurring on either side of the centerline and not entering zone C is also an extremely unlikely occurrence when the process follows the normal distribution and signals an out-of-control condition.*
- The probability of having 15 or more consecutive points occurring outside zone C is also an extremely unlikely occurrence when the process follows the normal distribution and tells you that you have an out-of-control condition.

* This occurs when more than one process is being followed on the same chart, when using improper sampling techniques.

10

Design Transfer

WHAT IS DESIGN TRANSFER?

When design controls first made their appearance, many people looked at the section concerning design transfer and pointed to it as proof of the bureaucratic nature of the new regulation. What else would you do with a newly developed product but transfer it to production? The problem is that it's not what you do at this point in the development but how—and sometimes even when—you do it. The purpose of the design transfer phase is to make sure design outputs are adequately and correctly translated into production specifications.

CHECK YOUR ATTITUDE AT THE DOOR

We are sure that nothing we are about to say in this section applies to your company, but you know it happens at Company "AB," and of course everyone has heard of the internal competition at Corporation "BA"! Design transfer is probably the most obvious phase of the design control cycle, and that is the root of the problem. Senior management causes the other fundamental problem of internal competition whether it does it consciously or unconsciously.

If management does not have a sincere commitment to the design control process and the teamwork and high quality the process represents, then this transfer, while obvious, becomes the source of fundamental problems. If management believes that some level of internal competition between functional groups brings out the best in everybody, then no one should be surprised when the product that was developed and looked so good in clinical evaluations isn't quite the one that actually got launched and is in inventory. It may look the same and have the same components, but somehow it isn't quite what it was.

Don't blame this on the fact that the product inevitably loses a little when it gets into production. If the design control process was followed and management created a team that took possession of the device from beginning *through* production, then it will not have changed.

Poor transfer happens more often than you might think. One of the scenarios for this poor transfer often starts with manufacturing personnel and is tacitly agreed to by general management. If there is a process engineering presence in the company, it almost always happens. Management decides that the participation of manufacturing personnel on the design team needs to be either limited or, worse, not at all. The rationalization for this is usually something like, "We are working three shifts a day and overtime. Manufacturing people simply don't have the time, and the company can't afford to take them away from their jobs for a meeting. They're too critical!"*

During the design process the manufacturing people hear all sorts of things about the new product, and most of them are out of context. Sometimes design engineers ask them questions, by design engineers and a mental picture begins to form of a new product that will be difficult to integrate into manufacturing at best and a nightmare at worst. As time goes on the manufacturing people begin to form a defense against this new product that often takes the form of, "When it gets to manufacturing, we'll fix it."

Never happens, right? It happens. Here are two instances that really occurred. Both were at well-known and well-respected companies. In the first case, a device was developed in-house, and R & D entirely handled the technical side of the development. The manufacturing process was designed, debugged, and validated by process engineering. The product was virtually demanded by the customers, and so its success was guaranteed. The first manufacturing line was built in-house and tested, and the validation was without significant problems. The machine was transferred to the manufacturing plant. For a period of three weeks on-specification product was made while the manufacturing personnel were trained. Process engineering stayed with manufacturing and the product for the entire three-week period. After everyone signed off his or her approval, the process engineers left. Within one month of the transfer, all hell broke loose. A critical design dimensional specification could not be held and manufacturing sought approval to loosen the specification. When the original process design engineers went to the facility, the reason for the sudden inability to hold the specification was apparent.

* The other extreme is, "We have problems with costs and quality. Manufacturing people simply don't have the time, and the company can't afford to take them away from their jobs for a meeting. They're too critical!"

The manufacturing engineers had redesigned the production equipment to increase efficiency and save floor space.* In doing so they cut the framework of the machine to rearrange its components. From that point on, the warped frame made it impossible to hold the dimensional specification. In another instance an outside source designed and built the manufacturing process. The line was installed and validated. Everyone was in heaven except, as it turned out, some of the manufacturing people didn't like the design of the machine and thought they had a better idea. So the machine began to act erratically. The cause for this sudden erratic behavior in the process was that someone in the plant disconnected a circuit.† The people responsible for the sabotage said they knew the machine was no good and they hoped that when it failed they would get the chance to build their own.‡

How could this happen? The reason is simple really. The manufacturing people were never involved; there was no ownership of the product from their point of view. Whose fault was it? That answer is also simple. It was the fault of the senior managers. It was their responsibility to ensure quality. It was senior management's responsibility to build the team. And one more important point, although the two examples happened to put manufacturing folks in a poor light: It could and does happen with other disciplines also. Manufacturing was used as the example because they are the one's most often left out.

THE FDA AND DESIGN TRANSFER

The FDA says, "Each manufacturer shall establish and maintain procedures to ensure that the device design is correctly

---

* They had a legitimate floor space problem. Business was growing so fast there was no room.

† By the way, the cause was uncovered by SPC due to the peculiar nature of the out-of-specification data points. It told the engineers that someone either had changed the machine or was faking the data.

‡ Yes, they were terminated.

translated into production specifications" [21 CFR Part 820, Subpart C, Section 820.30(h)]. There is no point in beating this one to death. It's simple and concise.

DESIGN TRANSFER REQUIREMENTS

Before we move on, it seems appropriate to list the requirements for an effective design transfer. A typical material specification and its corresponding quality specification are shown in Appendices H and I.

- When the design is complete, the design specifications need to be transferred to manufacturing in the form of production specifications. As always, the system for the transfer needs to be defined and documented.
- Production specifications typically consist of written documents. These documents include
    - product and assembly drawings
    - material specifications
    - inspection (quality) and test specifications
    - manufacturing instructions
    - training materials
    - tooling drawings

In addition, all verification and validation activities should be completed and all appropriate personnel training conducted before initial production begins. It is also an ideal time for a design review to ensure that all aspects of the design process were reviewed and transferred correctly. Now the product is ready to launch.

11

Design Changes

THE PURPOSE OF DESIGN CHANGE CONTROL

Design change control is just one more effort to ensure the highest quality in the product development process. Anyone that has ever been intimately involved with the development of a medical device is aware of how many changes happen between the original concept and the product that finally reaches production. If we remember that design control is a cyclic process, then it is important to know where we've been. For one thing, knowing where we've been tells us where we are, which in turn tells us where we can go.

Just like the pitfalls that can occur during design transfer, similar events can happen if the design team does not have control of the changes that occur along the way. If an overzealous design engineer decides to change a dimension without telling anyone, and worse without noting the change, a disaster can occur. It happens and you know it. Remember the first law of design controls: Document everything.

The section on design changes in the quality system regulation is simply about documentation. It is the foundation of a good product development cycle and the cornerstone of design controls.

THE FDA AND DESIGN CHANGES

In another concise and clear paragraph, the FDA has this to say about the subject:

> Each manufacturer shall establish and maintain procedures for the identification, documentation, validation or where appropriate verification, review and approval of design changes before their implementation. [21 CFR Part 820, Subpart C, Section 820.30(i)]

DESIGN CHANGE REQUIREMENTS

Once you approve your initial design inputs for the design project, changes must be documented and controlled for the life of the product, not just during the design controls cycle. The system for making design changes needs to be defined and documented in a procedure. This system should address how changes are identified and documented and how it is determined whether verification and/or validation is necessary. The degree of design change control depends on the significance of the change and the risk presented by the device.

Changes need to be reviewed and approved by the same individuals or functions associated with the original design to ensure the device will continue to perform as intended. Design changes include

- Changes made to the device itself
- Labeling changes

REQUEST NUMBER ___ SHEET ___ OF ___
[REFER TO SOP 100-007 FILL IN ALL APPLICABLE BLANKS]
REQUEST DATE: _____ ORIGINATOR/REQUESTOR: __________________
DEPARTMENT MANAGER: ______________________________________
PRODUCTS AFFECTED:

DOCUMENTATION AFFECTED:
[ORIGINATOR AND THOSE APPROVING MUST CHECK ANY CHANGES CAUSED BY THIS REQUEST IN THEIR RESPECTIVE AREAS.]
☐ DEVIATION ☐ ENGINEERING DRAWING ☐ INTERIM SPECIFICATION
☐ LABEL TEXT SPECIFICATION ☐ MATERIAL SPECIFICATION
☐ MERCHANDISING NOTICE ☐ PRODUCT SPECIFICATION ☐ QA POLICY
☐ QA SPECIFICATION ☐ STANDARD OPERATING PROCEDURE ☐ FORM
☐ OTHER: ________ [e.g., DMR, technical file, quality plan, 510(k) file note, etc.]
REQUEST TYPE:
☐ Document change/revision ☐ New document ☐ Document obsolescence ☐ Other
EFFECT CODES: CHECK THE APPROPRIATE BOX (ES)
☐ Immediate – all units in receiving inspection ☐ Immediate – all new manufacturing
☐ Immediate – all units in process ☐ Immediate – all units in finished goods
☐ Immediate purchase – on receipt of materials ☐ As of approval / effective date
☐ Upon depletion of current stock ☐ Begin with (date or control #) _________
☐ End with (date or control #): ___________ ☐ Other: _____________________
MATERIAL DISPOSITION: CHECK THE APPROPRIATE BOX(ES)
☐ check here if not applicable ☐ Use up existing parts ☐ Use existing parts until new arrive, then scrap old parts
☐ Rework ☐ Scrap ☐ Other reason for change or release:

Describe change or release:

DOCUMENTS AFFECTED [USE ADDITIONAL PAGES IF NECESSARY]

Title	Number	Revision (Old)	Revision (New)	Assigned to:

Review and approvals: [Approve and review – if change causes other documents under your supervision to require revision, note above and assign task]

Department/Signature	Date	Department/Signature	Date
Technology:		Manufacturing:	
QA/RA:		Clinical Affairs:	
Engineering:		Finance:	
President		Sales:	

Figure 1 Documentation change request.

- Performance changes
- Packaging changes
- Changes resulting from complaints, etc.

When a change is made to a specification, method, or procedure, the manufacturer should evaluate whether the change requires the submission of a premarket notification or a supplement to a PMA. An evaluation of many small/minor changes should also be considered in the same light. Records of this evaluation and the results need to be maintained.

Companies are required to maintain a defined and documented design change procedure even if they have not completed any design projects or have no ongoing or planned design projects or changes. A design change procedure is shown in Appendix J.

THE DOCUMENT CHANGE REQUEST

The heart of controlling design changes is the *document change request* (DCR), shown in Figure 1. This simple form provides the necessary control by requiring the originator of any change to think about what he or she is doing and what other documents, specifications, and tests the change may affect. In addition, the people responsible for the various corporate functions must review the changes, add any resultant changes of which they may be aware, and affix their signature in approval.

By keeping a log of all the DCRs in a central location, duplication will be improbable and tracing the origins of the changes to any product can be accomplished.

12

The Design History File

WHY DO WE NEED A DESIGN HISTORY FILE?

The prime reason for the design history file is to provide a record or evidence of compliance with design control requirements. The design history file is the final section of the design control topics in the quality system regulation and is by far the most simple. As manufacturers of medical devices, we are required to keep a complete record of the development of every medical device developed under the design control system. The design history file may be defined as a compilation of the records (drawings, formulations, test methods, etc.) that describes the design history of the finished device.

Of course, there are other sound reasons to compile this historical record of the development beyond the regulatory requirement. Some of these are as follows:

- The historical record will allow subsequent development teams to take advantage of things that were discovered by studying objective records.
- Postdevelopment review of the records will provide a unique vantage point for the continuous improvement of the product development cycle in general.
- The design history file provides an excellent evidentiary source in the event of patent disputes.
- In the event of unanticipated future product problems or complaints, the device history file may provide a valuable resource for solving the problem.

THE FDA AND THE DESIGN HISTORY FILE

In its last words on design control, the FDA addresses the concept of the device history file:

> Each manufacturer shall establish and maintain a DHF for each type of device. The DHF shall contain or reference the records necessary to demonstrate that the design was developed in accordance with the approved design plan and the requirements of this part [21 CFR Part 820, Subpart C, Section 820.30(j)]

DESIGN HISTORY FILE REQUIREMENTS

A design history file needs to be maintained for each device a manufacturer develops. It contains the records necessary to *demonstrate* that the design was developed in accordance with the approved design plan and the established design controls. The elements of the design history file include

- The plan
- Design inputs
- Design outputs
- Design review records
- Verification records and methods
- Validation protocols and results

13

Questions to Expect in an Audit

AN AUDIT! NOW WHAT?

So you're about to be audited. What can you expect? First of all, if you've been doing everything correctly, there is not much to worry about. It will happen sooner or later. If things are running smoothly, you should have conducted several internal audits before the FDA shows up for its inspection.

THE FDA DESIGN CONTROLS INSPECTION OBJECTIVES

In the quality system inspection technique (QSIT) *Guide to Inspections of Quality Systems*,* the FDA lists the objectives regarding design controls. There are 15:

* August 1999.

1. Select a single design project. Note: If the project selected involves a device that contains software, consider reviewing the software's validation while proceeding through the assessment of the firm's design control system.
2. For the design project selected, verify that design control procedures that address the requirements of Section 820.30 of the regulation have been designed and documented.
3. Review the design plan for the selected project to understand the layout of the design and development activities including assigned responsibilities and interfaces. Note: Evaluate the firm's conduct of risk analysis while proceeding through the assessment of the firm's design control system.
4. Confirm that the design inputs were established.
5. Verify that the design outputs essential for the proper functioning of the device were identified.
6. Confirm that the acceptance criteria were established prior to the performance of verification and validation activities.
7. Determine if the design verification confirmed that the design outputs met the design input requirements.
8. Confirm that the design validation data shows that the approved design met the predetermined user needs and intended uses.
9. Confirm that the completed design validation did not leave any unresolved discrepancies.
10. If the device contains software, confirm that the software was validated.
11. Confirm that risk analysis was performed.
12. Determine if design validation was accomplished using initial production devices or their equivalents.
13. Confirm that the changes were controlled including validation or, where appropriate, verification.
14. Determine if design reviews were conducted.
15. Determine if the design was correctly transferred.

SOME QUESTIONS YOU MAY BE ASKED

In addition to the material mentioned above, there are some questions that may arise during an audit.

General Design Controls

- What initiates a design project?
- When does the actual design and development begin (e.g., design controls)?

Design and Development Planning

- How is each design and development activity identified and documented?
- How are responsibilities defined?
- Are design and development activities assigned to qualified personnel?
- Are plans updated as the design evolves?
- Are the organizational and technical interfaces between different groups that input into the design process identified?
- Do procedures exist for the documentation, transmittal, and review of interdepartmental data exchanges?

Design Input

- Do design inputs include customer requirements?
- Do design inputs include applicable statutory and regulatory requirements for those countries in which you are intending to market?
- Do design inputs address intended uses, including the needs of the user and the patient?
- Are design inputs reviewed and approved?
- Does the company have a procedure/method to address incomplete, ambiguous, or conflicting requirements with those responsible for imposing these requirements?

Design Output

- Is design output documented and expressed in terms that can be verified and validated against design input requirements?
- Are design outputs approved?
- Does design output documentation
  - provide evidence that the final design meets input requirements?
  - identify or make reference to acceptance criteria?
  - identify characteristics of the design that are crucial to the safe and proper functioning of the product (for example, operating, handling, maintenance, storage, and disposal requirements)?

Design Review

- At what stages are formal documented reviews performed?
- Do design reviews include representatives of all functions concerned with the design stage being reviewed as well as an individual independent of the design stage being reviewed?
- Are records of design reviews maintained? If so, for how long?
- Do records include individuals in attendance, date, design reviewed?
- Do design reviews address, as applicable,
  - comparison of customer needs with technical specifications for materials, products, and processes?
  - validation of the design through prototype tests?
  - considerations of unintended use and misuse?
  - safety and environmental compatibility?
  - compliance with regulatory requirements, national and international standards, and corporate practices?
  - comparison with similar designs, especially analy-

  sis of internal and external problem history to avoid repeating problems?
  - permissible tolerances and comparison with process capabilities?
  - product acceptance/rejection criteria?
  - manufacturability of the design, including special process needs, mechanization, automation, assembly, and installation of components?
  - capability to inspect and test the design, including special inspections and test requirements?
  - specification of materials, components, and subassemblies, including approved suppliers?
  - packaging, handling, storage, and shelf-life requirements?
  - safety factors relating to incoming and outgoing items?
- How are problems or action items identified during a review handled?

Design Verification

- Do verification activities identify the method, date, and individual performing verification?
- What types of design verification activities were performed?

Design Validation

- What methods were used to validate the design?
- Were the first three production lots tested under actual or simulated use conditions?
- If design validation is done on nonproduction devices, how were the devices shown to be equal to production devices?
- How were unresolved discrepancies handled?
- If the device has software, how was the software validated?

Design Reviews

- Are there alternative calculations to verify the correctness of original calculations and analysis (i.e., risk assessment, AMPE, etc.)?
- Are there experimental runs?
- Are there tests and demonstrations (model or prototype test)?
- Is there a comparison to similar proven designs?
- Are design verification records maintained as part of the design history file?
- If output ≠ input, how was discrepancy resolved?

Design Transfer

- How are design specifications translated into production specifications?

Design Changes

- When do changes to product design begin to fall under design control?
- How are design changes controlled?
- Are all design changes identified, documented, reviewed, and approved by authorized personnel prior to implementation?
- Are design changes under document control?
- How do design changes trace back to the initial design project?

Design History File

- What documents make up your design history file?

Further Reading

Anderson, M.J. and P.J. Andrews, Design of experiments for process validation, *Medical Device & Diagnostic Industry*, Jan. 1999, 193–199.

ANSI/ASQC D1160-1995, Formal design review.

Augustine, R., A structural approach to rapid process development and control, *Medical Device & Diagnostic Industry*, Jan. 2000, 112–127.

Design control guidance for medical device manufacturers, FDA, 1997.

Dzog, H., Risk management in medical device regulations, *Medical Device & Diagnostic Industry*, Oct. 1997, 112–117.

Edwards, F., Before design, thoroughly evaluate your concept, *Medical Device & Diagnostic Industry,* Mar. 1997, 46–50.

FDA design input guidance, *The Silver Sheet*, June 1997, 11–14.

Federal Register, 21 CFR Part 820, 1996.

Final Q.C. inspectional strategy, CDRH, February 1998, 1–10.

Fleischer, M. and J.K. Liker, *Concurrent Engineering Effectiveness*, Hanser-Gardner, Cincinnati, 1997.

Giantini, R.E., Developing safe reliable medical devices, *Medical Device & Diagnostic Industry,* Oct. 2000, 60–67.

Goldratt, E.M. and J. Cox, *The Goal: Excellence in Manufacturing,* North River Press, New York, 1984.

Gosbee, J., The discovery phase of medical device design, *Medical Device & Diagnostic Industry*, Nov. 1997, 79–82.

Guide to inspections of quality systems, FDA, Aug. 1999.

Knepel, P., Integrating risk management with design controls, *Medical Device & Diagnostic Industry*, Oct. 1998, 83–88.

Kuhn, M.A., Implementing design controls, *Medical Device & Diagnostic Industry*, Feb. 2000, 40–49.

McCay, B., Design control measures that can boost return on investment, *Medical Device & Diagnostic Industry,* May 1998, 158–164.

Meyers, S.L., *Data Analysis for Scientists and Engineers*, Wiley & Sons, New York, 1975.

Munro, B.H., *Statistical Methods for Health Care Research*, Lippincott, New York, 1997.

Oliveri, D., Developing design control strategies to meet technology advances, *Medical Device & Diagnostic Industry*, Sept. 2000, 77–85.

Reich, R., How design controls affect sterilization process development & validation, *Medical Device & Diagnostic Industry*, Oct. 1997, 107–111.

Rubin, I.I., Product design, *Plastics Engineering*, April 2000, 101–106.

Sheratt, D., Taking a risk based approach to medical device development, *Medical Device & Diagnostic Industry*, Sept. 1999, 84–95.

Teixeira, M.B., *Design Controls Training Module*, QARA Compliance Connection, Odessa, NY, 2000.

Appendix A

Implementation Procedure

Rev. DCR*	Date	Effective Date	Originator	Description
A	07-20-98	08-14-98	M. Teixeira	DCR 98-0131

Approval signature: ____________________ Date: ____________

PURPOSE

The requirement to initiate a design control project may arise for a variety of reasons such as the identification of a new product, a marketing need to satisfy a customer's request/problem, a cost savings to the customer or company, the potential for a

* Document change request.

process improvement, or a change that is imposed by external circumstances. In all cases, the design control process is to be carried out under controlled conditions.

The purpose of this procedure is to define the system for controlling the design control process at Any Company, Inc., in order to ensure that specified design requirements are understood and met.

SCOPE

This procedure applies to all products developed by or for Any Company, Inc., that are required by the FDA Quality System Regulation to meet design control requirements.

DEFINITIONS

Design control project: a self-contained program of work initiated to either introduce a new product or process or to make a change to an existing product or process that may require redevelopment of that product or process.

Design history file: a compilation of records (drawings, formulations, test methods, etc.) that describes the design history of a finished device.

Design input: the physical and performance requirements of a device that are used as a basis for device design.

Design output: the results of a design effort at each design phase and at the end of the total design effort. The finished design output is the basis for the device master record. The total finished design output consists of the device, its packaging and labeling, and the device master record. Design outputs include the tests/procedures, etc. that are developed/utilized to show/meet the design input requirements.

Design review: a documented, comprehensive, systematic examination of a design to evaluate the adequacy of the design requirements, to evaluate the capability of the design to meet these requirements, and to identify problems.

Design validation: establishing by objective evidence that device specifications conform to user needs and intended use(s). (This may include laboratory testing.)

Design verification: a confirmation by examination and provision of objective evidence that specified requirements have been fulfilled and to what extent they have been achieved.

Human volunteer study: a study in which a test article is used on human volunteers to assess efficacy or user acceptance of the test article. The study may also yield limited information regarding test article safety; however, it is not performed to obtain such data.

Healthy human volunteer study: a product evaluation performed on volunteers that are usually in-house (laboratory based) and generally not suffering from the condition for which the device is intended to treat.

Clinical study: a product evaluation performed on patient volunteers.

Marketing evaluation (consumer preference test or field test): a study in which a marketed or nonmarketed test article is not used on humans but instead gathers input from humans, to assess physical and chemical characteristics of the test article; or a study in which a marketed test article is used on humans, but no individual medical data is collected (e.g., questionnaire).

Preliminary evaluation: work done to establish the basic merit of an idea.

Product evaluation: study designed to assess effectiveness and/or user acceptance of a product or intermediate (test article). These studies are usually *in-vivo* based, and performed on humans.

RESPONSIBILITIES

The R&D Department is responsible for planning, organizing, and managing design control projects. Project team members are responsible for acting as department liaisons in support of project requirements. Management is responsible for adhering to the requirements of this procedure and ensuring that employees comply. The project team leader is responsible for coordinating all aspects of the design control project.

REQUIRED EQUIPMENT

N/A

MATERIALS

N/A

RECORDS

Product initiation request (PIR)
Product performance specification (PPS)
Project design change form
Risk analysis master record (RAMR)
Design review meeting record
Design project plan
Meeting minutes comment form
Approval for sale

REFERENCES

Record retention
Project planning software or equivalent manual calculations
Risk analysis
Engineering change notice procedure
Document control procedure

PROCEDURE

There are typically four phases of any design control project:

Preliminary evaluation phase
Feasibility phase
Development/manufacture phase
Market introduction phase

Preliminary Evaluation Phase

As previously discussed, the requirement to initiate a design control project may arise for a variety of reasons and from a number of sources. Any offered products/technology or ideas may have some preliminary work performed to establish the basic merit of the idea, that is, a preliminary evaluation.

Feasibility Phase

If an idea appears to have merit, a product initiation request (PIR) shall be initiated to begin the feasibility phase. The Marketing Department is responsible for initiating the product initiation request. The PIR defines the basic requirements for a product and serves as the input for the feasibility phase. Any results of a preliminary evaluation should be incorporated into the PIR. Marketing should meet with the Technology Department to determine the feasibility of the requirements and the proper nomenclature.

The PIR form shall document the preliminary requirements. The following requirements shall be established (Note: A distinction should be made between desirable attributes and essential requirements):

Purpose/indication: Why develop product? What are the estimated market size and the potential exploitation/impact?

Market position: How is product to compete, against whom, and where?
Product: Essential and/or desirable requirements and parameters; for example:
delivery system
compatibility
sterilization requirements
preferred physical attributes (size, shape, color)
Claims: Those required to successfully and competitively market the product.
Packaging.
Clinical/technical.
Product costs (target).

Project team members shall be involved as necessary during the feasibility stage to support or offer other inputs and requirements; for example, regulatory, environmental, performance, labeling, etc.

Once the feasibility work is completed—that is, it is felt there is a viable product capable of meeting basic requirements—a report of the feasibility results (i.e., PPS, inclusive of financial information) will be generated and the project leader will call a formal design review meeting.

Development/Manufacture/First Clinical Use (Start of Formal Design Control) Phase

At the completion of the feasibility phase, the project leader is responsible for completing the PPS with assistance from other project team members as needed. The PPS serves as an output from the feasibility phase and as a primary input for the development/manufacture phase. The PPS shall document the product requirements. Any necessary changes regarding initial design inputs/outputs identified on the PIR shall be incorporated into the PPS. All inputs defined by the PPS shall be verifiable/quantifiable where possible, and any essential outputs for a device to ensure its proper performance, functioning, or use shall be defined. (Note: A distinction should be made between desirable attributes and essential requirements. Layman terms should be used. Customer expectations, safety, and satisfaction must be taken into consideration. If certain requirements are unique for a market, such as the European Community, then it should be indicated as such within the appropriate section. Additional description areas may be added as required.)

The PPS shall define the following:

Performance characteristics:

- indications for use of product
- clinical procedure for use
- relevant setting/use environment (e.g., nursing home, home care, hospital)
- medical specialty of user (e.g., doctor, nurse, end user/layperson)
- patient population inclusion/exclusion criteria
- clinical outcomes analysis (trial data)

Product characteristics

- Physical characteristics (e.g., dimensional, color, etc.)
- chemical characteristics (describe the direct chemical interactions of the product in preparation for and during a procedure, e.g., drugs, wipe downs, if applicable)
- biological characteristics (indicate the maximum duration of product use *in-vivo* (wear time) and body fluids and tissue to which the item will be exposed and toxicity and biocompatibility requirements)
- environmental characteristics (describe anticipated conditions in transportation, storage, and use, e.g., temperature, humidity, and/or any limitations, etc.)
- sterilization characteristics [describe the type of sterilization to which the product will be exposed

and the number of resterilization (dose) the product must be able to withstand]

- packaging (describe the packaging material and configuration in which the product will be sterilized and/or shipped)
- equipment interface (describe any accessories necessary for use of the product/device)
- safety and reliability requirements

Marketing requirements

- intended marketplace (United States, Europe, etc.)
- labeling (precautions, warnings, or contraindications)

Claims

Regulatory/quality assurance requirements

- relevant regulatory or statutory requirements [e.g., standards/test methods: FDA QSR, ISO 9001, EN 46001, 93/42/EEC (CE Mark), ASTM, etc.]

Financial requirements

- The market in which the product/device is to perform and market's size
- cost projection
- competitive environment (e.g., competitors, strengths, and weaknesses)
- proposed forecast/profit
- capital projection
- percent share of market (estimated shares)
- total opportunity
- resource assessment (engineering, packaging, regulatory, etc.)

The PPS shall be reviewed and approved by all project team members as part of the initial design review. Changes from this point forward shall be documented and controlled using the project design change form.

The project leader, or designee, shall create a project plan using standard off-the-shelf project planning software to define project tasks and activities, associated timeframes, and project team member/department responsibilities and interrelationships. The detail in which planning is carried out and documented may vary depending on the complexity and timescale of the project. All project team members shall approve the project plan as part of the initial design review. Project plans shall be reviewed, updated, and approved as the project evolves.

A risk analysis shall be conducted at the initial design review meeting in order to assess the risks and hazards associated with the use of a device/product. The risk analysis master record (RAMR) shall be approved by all project team members as part of the initial design review. The RAMR shall be reviewed at each subsequent design review.

Formal design review meetings shall be conducted at significant milestones to verify and/or validate that design outputs meet design input requirements. At a minimum, design reviews shall occur at the end of feasibility, the end of development, and prior to market introduction/product launch.

The purposes of the initial design review meeting are to formally define and confirm the design inputs and expected outputs and to initiate the development/manufacture phase. The PPS shall be a critical element of the initial design review. The initial design review meeting shall also formally define the design project team. All members must be present at the initial design review meeting, and each design review shall (1) consist of an individual who does not have direct responsibility for the design stage being reviewed and (2) include any specialists needed. Design reviews may include the review of design verification data to determine whether (1) the design outputs meet functional and operational requirements, (2) the design is compatible with components, (3) the safety requirements are achieved, (4) reliability and maintenance requirements are met, (5) labeling and other regulatory requirements are met, and (6) the manufacturing process is compatible with design specifications.

The initial design review meeting will review the design inputs, the expected outputs, and any known outcomes. The project plan, risk analysis, PPS, and any other pertinent information shall be included in the design review. The following format will be used to document design review meetings (design review meeting record). (Note: All inputs should be expressed in verifiable/quantifiable terms. Outputs should allow for an adequate evaluation/verification of conformance to design input requirements. As such, outputs should contain or make reference to acceptance criteria and identify characteristics of the design that are crucial to the safe and proper functioning of the product.)

Inputs	**Outputs**	**Review/Results**
(Inputs = outputs) *Requirement*	*Specification / test*	*(Verification / validation)* *Outcome*
Noncytotoxic	Agar diffusion method	Cytotoxicity report—Pass
Product sizes	Product specification	Inspection—Pass
Flow rate	Test method	Test—Pass
Wear time	Clinical protocol	Clinical study report
Expiration date	Stability protocol	Stability report
Package integrity	ASTM method	Transit trial report
CE mark	Declaration of conformity	CE technical file
Prescription	Product labeling	510(k)

Any incomplete, ambiguous, or conflicting requirements shall be resolved and documented as part of the design review meeting record.

A design review meeting record shall be generated to document the results of design review meetings.

If it is determined at the design review meeting that the product is not viable, not cost-effective, etc., the design project will be terminated. All associated data shall be retained in accordance with the record retention procedure. If the team decides to move forward with the design project, the design review meeting record shall be approved by all project team members. This will formally signify the initiation of the development/manufacture phase and the implementation of compliance with design controls.

The project team leader shall call project team meetings as necessary as inputs evolve and the project moves forward. Prior to each meeting an agenda will be issued that identifies topics of discussion and project team members required in attendance. The project leader or designee will record all design project meeting proceedings in minutes. The minutes will include copies of all tests or reports presented at that meeting. Project team members shall sign off on the minutes as to their agreement or disagreement by way of the meeting minutes comment form.

Any changes or conflicting, ambiguous, or incomplete requirements shall be addressed formally at the subsequent design review meeting.

As the design evolves in the development cycle, various methods of verification shall be used to determine whether the design outputs meet functional and operational requirements or design inputs. Design verification shall be performed on prototypes. Verification may be accomplished via a variety of methods, including design reviews, inspection/testing under simulated use conditions (i.e., *in-vivo* testing), biocompatibility testing, package integrity tests, risk analysis, comparison to similar designs [510(k)s], tests, and demonstrations, etc. Verification activities shall identify the method of verification, the date, and the individual performing the verification.

The project team leader shall call a design review meeting after development and verification of prototypes. Any changes that need to be implemented shall be documented and approved by all project team members on the design review meeting record. Manufacture of product under simulated use conditions (production runs) shall then commence.

Validation shall be performed under defined operating conditions on initial production lots. Design validation is performed to ensure devices conform to defined user needs and includes testing of production units under actual or simulated use conditions. The results of all validation activities shall include the identification of the design, the method(s), the date, and the individual performing the validation. Validation activities may include stability studies, validation (process/product), clinical evaluation, clinical studies, literature studies—(i.e., published journal articles), 510(k) comparison, transit trial, product/market evaluation, review of labels/labeling, etc. [Note: Process and/or product validation is a critical element of design control. Process/product validations are performed to validate production processes, for example, that manufacturing standard operating procedures (output) meet input requirements.]

Market Introduction

After all verification and validation activities have been completed, the project team leader shall call a final design review meeting. This meeting is the final confirmation that the overall design output has met the overall design input. All project team members are required at the final design review meeting. Any changes or conflicting, ambiguous, or incomplete requirements shall be documented on the design review meeting record, which shall be reviewed and approved by all project team members.

The final design review meeting shall include a final review of the risk analysis to assess any additional potential hazards associated with the device under normal and fault conditions. The risk analysis master record shall be updated and approved by all participating project team members. Any necessary changes shall be implemented prior to transferring design and development specifications/procedures to production specifications/procedures and sign-off of the approval for sale form.

Design Transfer

Transfer of product development specifications/procedures to production specifications/procedures shall be done using a document change request form in accordance with the document control procedure. Any required training shall be conducted and documented.

Approval for Sale

An approval for sale form is completed prior to product launch. The purpose of the approval for sale form is to document the confirmation from all project team members that all documents and data pertinent to their area(s) of responsibility and necessary to ensure that the product is ready for distribution are in place. The approval for sale form shall indicate in what countries the product has been approved for sale and at what price.

Design History File

A design history file (DHF) shall be established and maintained for each type of device. The DHF shall contain or reference the location of all documents/records needed to demonstrate compliance with the design plan and design control requirements. The elements of the DHF shall include, as applicable, the PIR, PPS, feasibility report, project team meeting minute and comment forms, design review meeting records, project design change forms, risk analysis master record, drawings/formulations, product development specifications/procedures, clinical testing, stability studies, project plans, safety testing, market evaluations, validations, transit trials, and approval for sale. The DHF shall be retained in accordance with the record retention procedure.

Design Changes

Any changes after the design has been transferred to Manufacturing shall be in accordance with the engineering change notice procedure.

Appendix B

Concept Document

PRODUCT INITIATION REQUEST

Product name: New Product X

Purpose/intended use: New Product X is a family of products intended to hermetically cover a site and apply healing entities at the site. New Product X also acts as a device that protects these sites from external contaminants. Intended launch is Quarter 1 2001.

Marketing position: (Check One)

Is product intended to be sold into the European Union as a medical device?

YES X No __

New Product X is intended for sale initially in the United States and Canada. It is recommended that all issues be addressed for sale of the product line in the European Union. By providing regulatory compliance for entry into the European Union from the outset, product components, design, packaging, and clinical research will be in place to take advantage of worldwide licensing opportunities. The device will be positioned as an adjunct therapy in whatever management and treatment and for the protection of various sites. In some market segments as, for example, prepackaged kits, the product will be offered to manufacturers of such products as an OEM product. The device will be positioned as a "positive management entity."

Product: Various sizes are planned, each with its own special adaptations for a particular market segment. This is a new indication for a class III device already approved.

INDICATIONS

U.S. marketed product: New Product X: A protective device for certain sites that provides a physical barrier to external contaminants.

European Union marketed product, if applicable: The same claims as in the United States.

Packaging: Sterile, single-unit, blister pack.

Clinical/technical: Initial clinical trial for safety and efficacy has been completed. Demonstration of positive patient management compared with competitor A and wear time have been completed.

Product Cost: Depending on product size and complexity of catheter connection, a direct manufacturing cost of between $X.XX and $X.XX for should be targeted.

SIGNATURE OF AUTHOR(S):

______________________ DATE: _____________

Appendix C

Product Specification

PRODUCT PERFORMANCE SPECIFICATION

Product name: New Product X

General description of product or system: New Product X is a family of products intended to hermetically cover a site and apply a therapeutic entity at a flow rate of about 1 liter per minute. The New Product X device is a derivative design of commercial product A, approved for marketing as a class III device indicated for the treatment of indication F, indication G, and indication H. New Product X is additionally designed as a device that protects these indications from external or environmental contaminants.

REVISION NUMBER: 0700-B

AUTHOR(S): ____________________ DATE: ______________

APPROVALS:

VP R&D:

____

VP Regulatory Affairs:

____

VP Sales and Marketing:

____

VP Manufacturing:

____

President/CEO:

____

Product Performance Specification (cont.)

I. Performance definitions: Distinction should be made between attributes and essential requirements. Layman terms should be used. Customer expectations, safety, and satisfaction must be taken into consideration. If certain requirements are unique for a market (e.g. Europe), then it should be indicated as such within the appropriate section. Additional description areas may be added as required.

Clinical Terms

Indications for Use of Product

New Product X [general]: indications F, G, and H; plus use as a protective device for these sites.

New Product X: indicated for use as a protective device over specific location. Provides all the benefits listed in the filing for Product A and provides a protective entity around the indication that protects the site from environmental contaminants.

Clinical Procedure for Use

Refer to instructions for use for Product A. The instructions (current revision) for use for New Product X are also included in this PPS by reference.

Relevant Setting/Use Environment (e.g., nursing home, home care, hospital)

Acute-care hospital, trauma centers, skilled nursing facility, chronic care settings, hospice, and home health care.

Medical Specialty of User (e.g., Doctor, Nurse, End User/Layperson)

Nurse, doctor, and home health care provider.

Patient Population Inclusion/Exclusion Criteria

Excludes all patients allergic to the ingredients or components of the product and patients excluded from using Product A. It is expected that New Product X would continue to be "for sale by or on the order of a physician." It would remain a prescription product.

Clinical Outcomes Analysis (Trial Data)

Initial safety and efficacy. Initial safety and efficacy testing was included in the filing for Product A. The components of New Product X are similar, if not identical. A Phase 1 clinical study on the wear time, ease of use, and patient comfort levels is underway and the results will be used for any necessary design changes. The results of the trial are expected to be completed by (date), and will be kept on file.

Product Characteristics

Physical Characteristics (Dimensional, Color, etc.)

New Product X comes in various sizes and model types depending on the specific application/use. It is a sterile, single-use, disposable device. In general, it will be rectangular with rounded corners. A specific medical pressure-sensitive adhesive is used to anchor the device to the skin. Six medical-grade polyurethane tubes are attached. Four are inlet and outlet tubes for the introduction of the protective entity into and out of the device. The remaining two tubes are for the connection through the device into the indication. All tubes have a plastic clip to control flow through the tubes. The New Product X device has a clear, see-through polyurethane bubble that allows the clinician an unobstructed view of the site and areas adjacent to the indication.

The initial product will have overall rectangular dimensions of 25.50″ length by 22.25″ width. The four corners of the rectangle will be rounded to a radius of 2 in. There will be an adhesive border with a 5.5″ width on the outside perimeter of the product. The adhesive side mounts toward the body and anchors the device in place on the patient. The center of the rectangle that becomes the working area has dimensions of

15.0″ × 12.75″. Six polyurethane tubes are attached to the chamber. Four are the inlet and outlet tubes for the introduction of the protective entity into and out of the device. These two tubes are approximately 16″ to 17″ long and have a 0.175″ outside diameter and a 0.125″ inside diameter. Each has a clip for closing that tube. The two remaining tubes are for the connection of the device into the indication. This tube is 10″ to 12″ long (with 4″ to 5″ remaining inside the device and 6″ to 7″ of its length outside the device). This tube has an inside diameter of 0.125″ and an outside diameter of 0.175″. It also has a pinch clip to shut off flow through the tube. The distal end of this tube is terminated in a male Luer lock, while the proximal end is terminated in a female Luer lock connector with a male lock cap. A product drawing LTS 091300-00 is attached.

Chemical Characteristics (Describe the Direct Chemical Interactions of the Product in Preparation for and During a Procedure, e.g., Drugs, Wipe Downs, if applicable)

Formulation of the adhesive barrier must be able to withstand the presence of IPA and other liquids and materials found in hospitals. Operates with material XX. Suitable operating pressure will be determined by *in-vitro* and *in-vivo* testing. Clinical testing to date indicates that a flow rate of 1 l/min is sufficient to keep the device operational.

Biological Characteristics [Indicate the Maximum Duration of Product Use *in-Vivo* (Wear Time), Body Fluids and Tissue to Which the Item Will Be Exposed, and Toxicity and Biocompatibility Requirements]

Product will be replaced every 3 to 5 days or when it is necessary for the health-care professional to have access to the indication. It will generally be placed on intact, dry skin. Several devices may be used for several weeks and could possibly be used up to 30 days. The device should not be in direct contact with circulating blood. All components contacting the patient should be nonirritating, noncytotoxic, and hypoallergenic. Data included with the original filing indicates that the components meet these criteria. Data on alternative materials, if any, will be received from the manufacturer prior to use.

The components that would normally contact the skin would be the medical-grade adhesive, the connectors on the centerline attachment, and the tubing of the centerline attachment. It is possible that in the event of a failure to maintain sufficient operating conditions that the device film could also contact the patient.

One suitable adhesive is manufactured by XX and converted by YY. Their tape is essentially polyethylene film coated on both sides with a hypoallergenic pressure-sensitive acrylate adhesive. It is supplied on a paper liner, which is bleached and silicone-coated on both sides. XX has certified the safe and effective use of its No. 575783 Medical Tape for its intended use. Biocompatibility tests completed include *in-vitro* cytotoxicity (agar overlay), *in-vitro* hemolysis, acute primary skin irritation in albino rabbits, repeated insult patch (Draize) in humans, 21-day cumulative irritation in humans, intracutaneous irritation in albino rabbits, and acute systemic toxicity in mice.

Suitable polymer, for both tubing and molded connectors, is supplied by TT Compounds, a subsidiary of ZZZ. Testing from NAMSA on plaques included acute systemic toxicity, intracutaneous toxicity, and implantation test. This data is on file at Any Company, WWW Medical (contract manufacturer of New Product X prototypes), and at the manufacturer of the components. Material is class VI. This safety testing is also applicable to the polymer-molded connectors.

Input and output tubing is medical-grade polyurethane with a Shore A hardness of 80, which is the same tubing used to manufacture Product A. This tubing may also be used for the other tubing. The device film is medical-grade polyurethane—Trademark 329480 or equivalent. Specifications are currently maintained at WWW Medical in City, State along with appropriate safety testing on urethane components. (tubing, film, and connectors) WW documentation 24185-6503391 Rev B. Transfer of documentation to Any Company is underway.

All fittings and connectors will be plastic and molded from acrylic, polycarbonate, nylon, or high-density polyethylene as received from the suppliers of these medical connectors and clamps. Safety data and certificates of compliance are on file. This data is in addition to the data cited above on the materials themselves.

Environmental Characteristics (Describe Anticipated Conditions in Transportation, Storage, and Use, e.g. Temperature, Humidity, and/or Any Limitations, etc.)

It is not anticipated that the product will be subjected to any unusual conditions in storage and/or transportation. During use the product must withstand a positive pressure of 10 cm (H_2O). Normal precautions must be taken with regard to operating. See Product A instructions for use. The adhesive has a 2-year shelf life and should be stored between 50° to 80° F at 40% to 60% humidity.

Sterilization Characteristics (Describe the Type of Sterilization to Which the Product Will Be Exposed and the Number of Resterilization (Dose) the Product Must Be Able to Withstand]

These are intended to be single-use products. New Product X will require gamma or electron-beam sterilization due to the nature of the materials. EtO will be excluded, as it will be impossible to remove this gas from the device.

Gamma sterilization should be anticipated at a dose of 2.5 MRad, with a sterility assurance level of 10^{-6}. Dosimetry is required at 3 MRad ± 10%. Sterility at a lower dose is possible, as is dosimetric sterility release, depending on the bioburden levels of the manufacturing facility.

Packaging (Describe the Packaging Material and Configuration in Which the Product Will Be Sterilized and/or Shipped)

Sterile, single-use, PETG blister packs with Tyvek® for each unit.

Equipment Interface (Describe Any Accessories Necessary for Use of the Product/Device)

N.A.

Safety and Reliability Requirements

Color-coded fittings will be used to differentiate the inlet and outlet tubes from the site line. Transparent tubes, film, and fittings are used to ensure visibility. Failure analysis will be conducted and documented on completion of first production run.

Marketing Requirements

Intended Marketplace

U.S. Market (Domestic): New Product X is expected to grow from $1.5 million in sales during the first full year of sales to $83.5 million in year 5.

International Market (List Countries): United Kingdom, Germany, Scandinavia, Italy, Belgium, Netherlands, France, and Spain.

Labeling (Precautions, Warnings, Contraindications): Currently as they appear in the instructions for use and/or product labeling.

Claims: New Product X: all claims of Product A plus use as a protective device for F, G, and H. The insert is attached. The device excludes external contaminants.

Regulatory/Quality Assurance Requirements

Relevant Regulatory or Statutory Requirements [e.g., Standards/Test Methods—FDA QSR, ISO 9001, EN 46001, 93/42/EEC (CE Mark), ASTM, etc.]

FDA 21 CFR Part 807: Device listing and establishment registration
FDA 21 CFR Part 820: FDA quality system regulation
EN 46001: Europe's QS requirements for medical devices
FDA 21 CFR Part 801: Labeling
FDA 21 CFR Part 803: Medical device reporting
MDD: Medical device vigilance requirements
FDA 21 CFR Parts 7: Recall/remedial action
FDA 21 CFR 806: Reports of corrections and removals
ISO 10993: Biocompatibility testing
93/42/EEC: Medical device directive
ANSI/AAMI/ISO 11037 or 11035: Sterilization (gamma or EtO)
EN 550: EtO
EN 552: Irradiation (gamma)
EN 554: Moist heat
EN 980 and EN 1041: Labeling
EN 556: Requirements for terminally sterilized devices to be labeled "sterile"
ISO 11067: Packaging for terminally sterilized medical devices
EN 868-1: General requirements and test methods—packaging materials and systems for medical devices, which are to be sterilized (this is a series of standards)
EN 1441: Risk analysis
PrEN 12442-1,2,3: Animal tissue materials
FDA Docket No. 98D-0924: Animal tissue materials
FDA validation guidance document
Validation of sterilization: AAMI/ISO 11137 Method 1

Package integrity: ASTM F88 seal strength; ASTM D1140 burst strength

ASTM Test Methods—Film: ASTM D638: Tensile properties; ASTM D1003: Test method for haze and luminous transmission of transparent plastic; ASTM D1004: Initial tear resistance; ASTM D1044: Resistance of transparent plastics to surface abrasion; ASTM D 1239: Resistance of plastic film to extraction by chemicals; ASTM D1709: Test method for impact resistance of film (falling dart); ASTM D2582: Puncture-propagation tear resistance of plastic film.

Adhesive: ASTM D896: Resistance of adhesive bonds to chemical reagents; ASTM D903: Peel strength; ASTM D1002: Shear strength; ASTM D1151: Effect of moisture and temperature on bond strength; ASTM D3121: Tack (rolling ball).

It may not be necessary to complete all these particular test methods; substitution by tests performed by the manufacturer of the components purchased by LifeTech may be sufficient. Quality test development should use these properties as a guide in determining testing of components and final product.

Financial Requirements

Market the Product/Device Is to Perform in and Size

The total market in the United States is $64 billion and growing at 16.4% per year.

Cost Projection

Total operating costs are approximately $3 million.

Competitive Environment (e.g., Competitors, Strengths, and Weaknesses)

A predicate device table is included with the FDA submission and is incorporated here by reference.

Proposed Forecast/Profit

See business plan.

Capital Projection

See business plan. Product will be produced at the Maui facility.

Percent Share of Market (Estimated Share)

Less than 5%.

Total Opportunity

Current estimate of market size is $14 billion.

Resource Assessment (Engineering, Packaging, Regulatory, etc.)

Will require the following:

- Design (product and process)
- Regulatory
- Clinical
- Sales and marketing
- Quality assurance/testing
- Reimbursement consultant
- Patent attorney
- Outside source

Appendix D

Product Claims Sheet

Product Name:	
Intended Use(s)	
Product Claims	
Claims	Supporting Data
Precautions and Warnings:	
Contraindications:	
Compiled By:	
Director Quality Assurance/ Regulatory Affairs Approval/Date:	
Director Sales and Marketing Approval/Date:	
Director Clinical Studies Approval/Date:	
Revision and Revision Date:	

Appendix E

Risk Analysis: Standard Operating Procedure

RISK ANALYSIS

Rev.	**DCR Date**	**Effective Date**	**Originator**	**Description**
A	04-02-00	04-27-00	M. Teixeira	DCR 00-0115

Approval Signature: ____________________ Date: __________

1.0 PURPOSE

1.1 Judgments relating to the safety, including the acceptability of risks, are necessary in order to determine the suitability for use of a product. Such judgments take into account the manufacturer's intended use; the performance, risks, and benefits of the product; and the risks and benefits associated with the clinical performance.

1.2 The criteria that must be evaluated/met regarding the safety, function, and quality of the product are as follows:

> The product must be designed and manufactured in such a way that, when used under the conditions and for the purpose intended, it will not compromise the clinical condition or the safety of the patients, or the safety and health of users or, where applicable, other persons, provided that any risks that may be associated with their use constitute acceptable risks when weighed against the benefits to the patient and are compatible with a high level of protection of health and safety.

This procedure outlines the requirements for performing a risk analysis assessment to investigate the safety of a product by identifying hazards and estimating the risks associated with the product.

2.0 SCOPE

2.1 This procedure applies to those individuals responsible for performing a risk analysis assessment in support of the CE mark or any other design control project.

3.0 DEFINITIONS

3.1 Harm: physical injury and/or damage to health or property

3.2 Hazard: a potential source of harm

3.3 Risk: the probable rate of occurrence of a hazard causing harm and the degree of severity of the harm

3.4 Risk analysis: the investigation of available information to identify hazards and to estimate risks

3.5 Safety: freedom from unacceptable risk of harm

4.0 RESPONSIBILITIES

4.1 Director of Quality Assurance and Regulatory Affairs: is responsible for coordinating the completion of the risk analysis, ensuring that all the necessary documentation is available, and arranging final review and approval of the risk analysis report.

5.0 REQUIRED EQUIPMENT

5.1 N/A

6.0 ASSOCIATED MATERIALS

6.1 N/A

7.0 RECORDS

7.1 Risk analysis master record

8.0 REFERENCES

8.1 Medical device directive (93/42/EEC)

8.2 EN 1441 Medical devices—risk analysis

8.3 Guide to identification of characteristics which could affect safety, Appendix I
8.4 Examples of possible hazards and contributing factors, Appendix II
8.5 SOP 100-003 Record retention
8.6 SOP 100-004 Complaint handling procedure
8.7 SOP 100-007 Document control
8.8 SOP 700-001 CE technical files
8.9 SOP 700-002 Medical device vigilance reporting
8.10 SOP 700-008 CE document control
8.11 Design control procedures (400 series)
8.12 Risk analysis master record
8.13 Risk analysis matrix

9.0 PROCEDURE

9.1 Once it has been determined that an existing device is to be CE marked or that a new product to be developed is to be CE marked, the hazards and risks associated with the use of the device/product need to be analyzed. A risk analysis shall be the method used to analyze and assess the device's risks and hazards. The risk analysis shall be performed by individuals from various departments (e.g., Technology, Mfg, Mktg, etc.).

9.2 For new products the risk analysis should be done after the feasibility stage. It should be updated as necessary, as the development process evolves.

9.3 Flow diagram of risk analysis procedure

9.4 Refer to the RAMR form

9.4.1 Heading: The heading of the RAMR contains the product name, product description, intended use, and the signatures of the individuals involved in the risk analysis process.

9.4.2 Characteristics that could affect safety: List

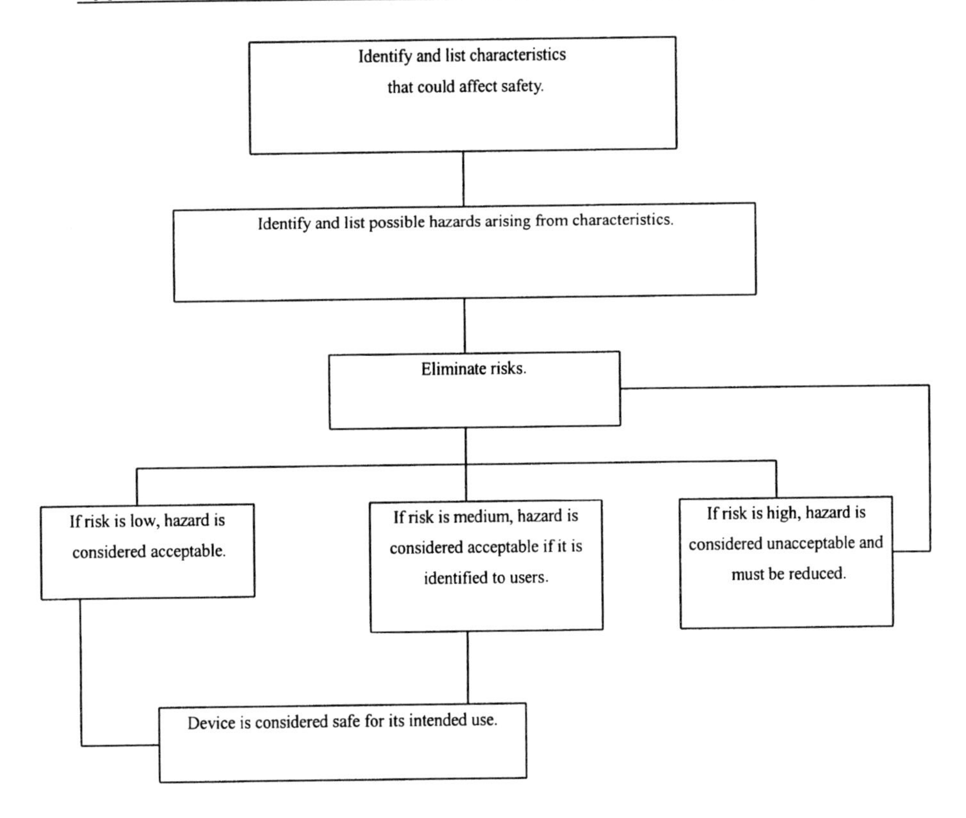

Figure 1 Carrying out the above procedure results in a risk analysis master record (RAMR).

all the characteristics that could affect the device's safety. A nonencompassing list, which can be used as a guide to identify characteristics, is given in Appendix I.

9.4.3 Possible hazard associated with characteristics: The hazard is a potential source of harm resulting from a characteristic that could affect safety. Compile a list of potential hazards associated with the device in both normal and fault conditions. A nonencompassing list of potential hazards is given in Appendix II.

9.4.4 Estimation of risks: For each possible hazard, estimate the associated risk(s) under both normal and fault conditions. Consider the implications (severity) of the hazard actually happening and the probability of the hazard occurring. To estimate the risks, refer to the risk assessment matrix.

Severity level:

- Catastrophic 1. Loss of life. Severe, permanent damage to health.
- Critical 2. Serious injury, possibly life threatening, but reversible. Requires medical intervention (e.g., severe burns).
- Marginal 3. Minor injury, but cause significant discomfort (e.g., minor burns).
- Negligible 4. Minor injury with minor discomfort, readily reversible.

In the column "Risk assessment," the resultant analysis should be in the format High/Medium/Low and indicate the probability/severity (e.g., Low (C4), Medium (E2), etc. derived from risk assessment matrix).

9.4.5 Acceptability of risk/risk reduction: If the risk is high (as determined on the risk assessment matrix), this is unacceptable and needs to be addressed. This unacceptable risk should be reduced to acceptable levels by appropriate means. Examples are given below.

- Direct safety means (design).
- Indirect safety means (safeguarding).

Examples of safeguarding are restricting accessibility (e.g., for radiation hazards) and shielding from the hazard (e.g., by means of a protective cover).

- Descriptive safety means (e.g., restricting period or frequency of use of the device, restricting application, lifetime, or environment).
- Redefining intended use.
- Record how the risk is addressed. If the risk is medium, it will commonly be addressed by warnings/instructions, etc. on the device packaging or the instruction leaflet. If the risk is low, it is optional whether warnings/instructions are provided. When possible, risks should be reduced or eliminated. When the risk has been identified as high, the risk should be reduced to acceptable levels.

9.4.6 Evaluations for new products/existing products: For existing products, perform a complaint review and a nonconformance review. The complaint review should consider how long the product has been on the market, the number of complaints on record, and the nature of these complaints. The nonconformance review should consider the nonconformances related to relevant product and any risk(s) associated with these nonconformances.

9.4.7 Comments: Indicate any additional comments here (e.g., product status with regards to the FDA, etc.).

9.4.8 Sign-off: Upon completion of the RAMR, the signature of the Director of Quality Assurance and Regulatory Affairs and the date are required.

9.4.9 Supporting documentation: All documentation supporting the risk analysis process will be attached to the RAMR.

9.4.10 Storage of risk analysis master records: RAMRs will be maintained in Regulatory Affairs. RAMRs will be retained according to appropriate procedure.

9.5 Amendments/changes to the RAMR

The RAMR may require amendment/change when:

- An additional indication/intended use is made for the product.
- Additional product codes are added to the product line.
- Changes are made to the product.
- Complaints are received on the product.
- New risks are identified (e.g., as a result of technology).
- A change in the device classification occurs.

The revision status and control of the RAMR is per applicable control procedure. The reason for change will be noted in the change history.

RISK ASSESSMENT MATRIX

SEVERITY

Catastrophic 1					
Critical 2		High		Medium	
Marginal 3					
Negligible 4				Low	
Probability	A Frequent	B Probable	C Occasional	D Remote	E Improbable

SUPPLEMENT 1 RISK ASSESSMENT SOP

Guide to Identification of Characteristics That Could Affect Safety

1. What is the intended use, and how is the device to be used?
2. Is the device intended to contact the patient or other persons?
3. What materials and/or components are incorporated in the device or are used?
4. Are substances delivered to and/or extracted from the patient?
5. Is the device supplied sterile or intended to be sterilized by the user, or are other microbiological controls applicable?
6. Is the device intended to modify the patient's environment?
7. Is the device intended to control or to interact with other devices or drugs?
8. Is the device susceptible to environmental influences?
9. Are there essential consumables or accessories associated with the device?
10. Does the device have a restricted shelf life?
11. Are there possible delayed and/or long-term use effects?
12. To what mechanical forces will the device be subjected?
13. What determines the lifetime of the device?
14. Is the device intended for single use or reuse?
15. Can the device be used by a high-risk patient (e.g., infant, elderly, immunocompromised, etc.)?
16. How is the device sold (e.g., sterile, nonsterile, preserved, etc.)?

SUPPLEMENT 2 RISK ANALYSIS SOP

Estimation of Toxicological Risk

The toxicological risk analysis should take account of

- The chemical nature of the materials
- The identity, concentration, availability, and toxicity of all constituents (e.g., additives, processing aids, monomers, catalysts, reaction products, etc.)
- The influence of biodegradation and corrosion on the material
- Prior use of the materials
- Biological safety test data

SUPPLEMENT 3 RISK ANALYSIS SOP

Examples of Possible Hazards and Contributing Factors

Environmental Hazards

- Likelihood of operation outside prescribed environmental conditions
- Incompatibility with other devices
- Accidental mechanical damage
- Contamination due to waste products and/or device disposal

Biological Hazards

- Bioburden
- Biocontamination
- Biocompatibility
- Incorrect formulation (chemical composition)
- Toxicity
- (Cross) infection
- Pyrogenicity
- Inability to maintain hygienic safety
- Degradation

Hazards Related to the Use of the Device

- Inadequate labeling
- Inadequate operating instructions
- Inadequate specification of accessories
- Inadequate specification of preuse checks
- Overcomplicated operating instructions
- Unavailable or separated operating instructions
- Use by unskilled/untrained personnel
- Reasonably foreseeable misuse
- Insufficient warning of side effects
- Inadequate warning of hazards likely with reuse of single-use devices
- Incompatibility with consumables/accessories/other devices

Hazards Arising from Functional Failure, Maintenance, and Aging

- Inadequacy of performance characteristics for the intended use
- Lack of adequate determination of end of device life
- Loss of mechanical integrity
- Inadequate packaging (contamination and/or deterioration of the device)

Appendix F

Cause-and-Effects Diagram

A cause-and-effects diagram illustrates the relationship between an outcome and all the factors that influence that outcome. Because of their shape, these diagrams have sometimes been called a "fishbone diagram."* The diagram is intended to show the relationship of the parts to the whole by

- Determining the factors that cause an outcome or effect, whether these factors are positive or negative

* The cause-and-effect diagram is also referred to as an "Ishikawa diagram."

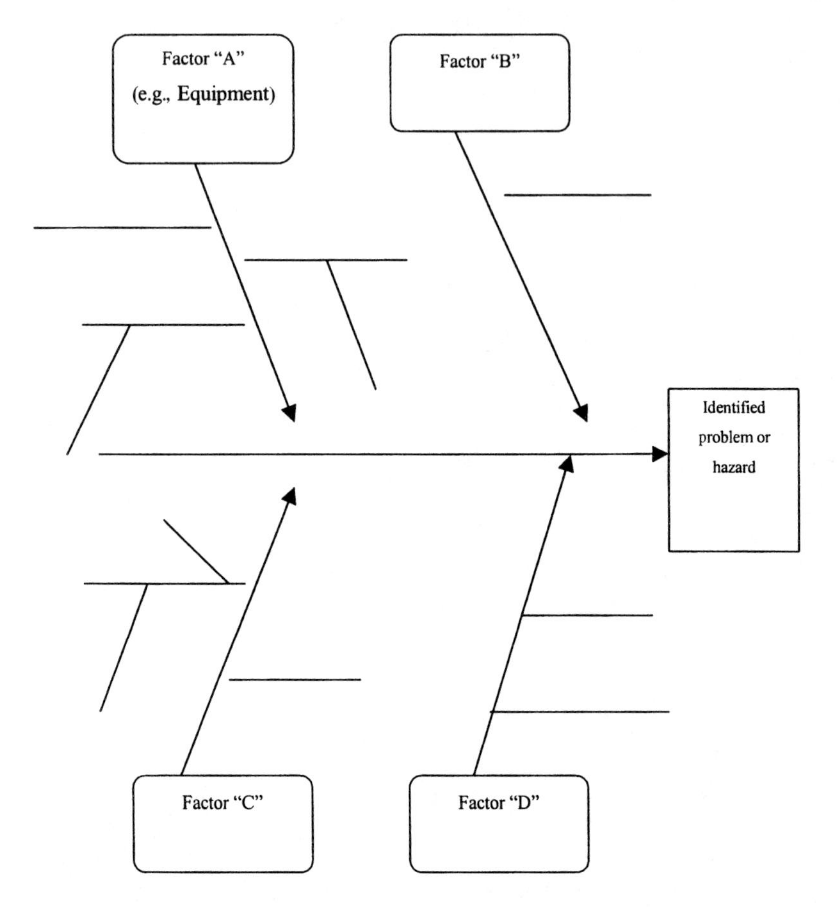

Figure 1 Typical cause-and-effect diagram.

- Focusing on a specific issue without resorting to irrelevant discussion*
- Determining the controllable cause of an effect
- Identifying areas in which there is inadequate or no objective data

* In this case irrelevant discussion is a polite way of saying complaining, blame shifting, and CYA activities.

The first step in preparing a cause-and-effect diagram is to specify what problem or hazard needs to be analyzed. This is placed in a box on the right side of the diagram. The second step is to list the major factors that influence the hazard being analyzed. These factors may include things like personnel, materials, components, process, machinery, maintenance, specifications, design flaws, etc. The next step is to identify subfactors within each of the major categories already identified. The final step is to prioritize the list of causes, that is, to identify which of the causes is the basis for the hazard. Keep in mind that the placement of a given cause on a diagram is not an indicator of its importance. The diagram should also help identify factors for which you may need to collect additional information, especially if one of the factors was not previously considering during the development.

Figure 1 is an example of a typical cause-and-effect diagram.

Appendix G

Validation Procedure

Rev.	DCR Date	Effective Date	Originator	Description
A	08-19-93		R. Bradley	Quality assurance policy
B	02-03-97	06-30-97	R. Bradley	Original release of policy
C	06-08-98	06-15-98	M. Teixeira	DCR 98-0094
D	08-18-98	08-28-98	M. Teixeira	DCR 98-0147

Approval Signature: ____________________ Date: __________

PURPOSE

To establish a documented procedure and process for obtaining, recording, and interpreting results required to show that a process will consistently produce a product that meets predetermined specifications.

SCOPE

This procedure applies to all products. The details and extent of process validation will vary depending on the nature of the device and the nature and complexity of the process being validated. Process validation covers three activities: qualification of process installation and setup; qualification of process capability; and process long-term stability (i.e., IQ, OQ, and PQ).

DEFINITIONS

Installation qualification: establishing by objective evidence that all key aspects of the process, process equipment, and ancillary system installation adhere to the approved design criteria and that the recommendations of the manufacturer of the equipment are suitably considered.

Operation qualification: establishing by objective evidence parameters that result in a product that meets all predetermined requirements.

Operating parameters: If the equipment being validated has variable control settings or parameters, the range over which the process can operate and produce within specified AQLs should be clearly stated. If the upper and lower process limits have been challenged by the protocol, the resulting parameters should be identified.

Performance qualification: establishing by objective evidence that the process, under anticipated conditions, including worst-case conditions, consistently produces a product that meets all predetermined requirements.

Process validation: establishing by objective evidence that the process consistently produces a result or product meeting its predetermined specifications.

Process validation protocol: a document stating how validation will be conducted, including test parameters, product characteristics, manufacturing equipment, and decision points on what constitutes acceptable test results.

Retrospective process validation: validation of a process for a product already in distribution based on accumulated production, testing, and control data.

Validation: confirmation by examination and provision of objective evidence that the particular requirements for a specific intended use are fulfilled.

Verification: confirmation by examination and provision of objective evidence that specified requirements have been fulfilled.

Worst case: a set of conditions encompassing upper and lower processing limits and circumstances, including those within standard operating procedures, that pose the greatest chance of process or product failure when compared to ideal conditions. Such conditions do no necessarily induce product or process failure.

RESPONSIBILITIES

The validation team has the responsibility for planning the validation approach and defining the requirements. The validation team may include representatives from or personnel with experience in Quality Assurance, Engineering, Manufacturing, Research and Development, Clinical Affairs, etc.

The Quality Assurance Department has the responsibility to prepare installation/operation and performance protocols and reports in accordance with this procedure and to provide technical support for process validations.

The Technology Department has the responsibility for assisting in defining and fulfilling the requirements of the installation/operation and performance qualification protocols (e.g., identifying operating parameters, determining/developing procedures, developing cleaning and maintenance and calibration requirements, etc.).

EQUIPMENT

N/A

MATERIALS

N/A

RECORDS

Validation risk assessment
Process validation decision tree
Installation qualification
Operation qualification
Performance qualification

REFERENCE

SOP 100-003 Record retention
SOP 700-005 Risk analysis
Global harmonization task force study group #3—"Draft process validation guidance"

PROCEDURE

General

Validation requires documented evidence that a process consistently conforms to requirements. It requires that you first establish a process that can consistently conform to requirements and that you then run studies demonstrating that this is the case. A number of statistical tools are available to aid in performing both of these tasks (e.g., acceptance sampling, FMEA, challenge tests, capability studies, etc.).

Those processes for which the product cannot be fully verified typically require that process validation be performed. As a guide, the process validation decision tree shall be used in determining whether or not a process should be validated.

Note: Each process should have a specification describing both the process parameters and the output desired. Consideration should then be given to whether the output can be verified by inspection and/or test (A). If the answer is positive, then the consideration should be made as to whether or not verification alone is a sufficient and cost-effective solution (B). If yes, the output should be verified and the process should be appropriately controlled (C). If the output of the process is not verifiable, then consideration with regard to the risk to the patient of the process or the final product (D) should be given. If the risk is high, then the decision should be to validate the process (G). If the risk is low, then justification for not validating the process should be considered (E). Consequently, management may decide to validate a process even though the output of the process is verifiable (F).

Processes that should normally be validated include

1. Sterilization processes
2. Clean-room ambient conditions
3. Sterile packaging sealing processes
4. Plastic injection molding processes

Processes that may be satisfactorily covered by verification include

1. Manual cutting procedures
2. Testing for color, turbidity, total pH
3. Visual inspection/testing of assemblies

Processes for which the decision tree may be useful in determining the need for validation include

1. Cleaning processes
2. Certain human assembly processes
3. Numerical control cutting processes

Note: Software utilized in manufacturing or testing processes should be validated for its intended use.

Determining the Need for Validation

Prior to the initiation or consideration of any process validation efforts of a new process or a product/process change, a validation risk assessment form shall be completed by the party/group proposing a new piece of equipment or a change.

As a minimum, the validation risk assessment should consider the following:

1. Impact on the product/process
2. Risk to the patient
3. Review of final product specifications
4. Review of machine design capability (i.e., is equipment properly designed to accomplish end goal?)
5. Equipment instrumentation and required calibration
6. Environmental considerations
7. Applicable procedures (e.g., process specifications, cleaning, maintenance, etc.)
8. Desired performance and quality parameters

As a minimum, the Vice President of Technology and the Director of Quality Assurance/Regulatory Affairs shall approve all validation risk assessment forms.

To determine the impact or risk to the patient, the risk analysis procedure should be referenced with regards to use of the risk analysis master record and the risk assessment matrix.

Once all applicable information has been delineated on the validation risk assessment form, the process validation decision tree (Appendix A) should be used to assist in determining if validation is required. If it is determined that no validation is required, the reason/justification for not doing so shall be documented on the validation risk assessment form and the form forwarded to Quality Assurance for filing. If a decision is made to validate, the validation risk assessment form should be used as a tool in developing the validation protocol(s).

Validation Protocol Generation

Detailed protocols for performing validations are essential to ensure that the process is adequately validated. A validation package shall contain, although *not* limited to, an installation qualification protocol and a performance qualification protocol.

For all phases of a process validation (IQ, OQ, PQ), the following should be determined:

1. What to verify/measure
2. How to verify/measure
3. How many to verify/measure (i.e., statistical significance)
4. When to verify/measure
5. Acceptance/rejection criteria
6. Required documentation

Validation Protocol Format

1. Title page.
2. Identify the process, product, or equipment undergoing validation/qualification.
3. Identify the author of the protocol.
4. Abstract—briefly describe the intent of the protocol [i.e., identification of device(s) to be manufactured using this process].

5. Protocol approval. Sign-off by Technology, Quality Assurance, and Manufacturing is required prior to performing the installation protocol.

Installation Qualification Protocol

1. Introduction
2. Objective
3. Scope/intended use
4. Applicable part numbers
5. Background
6. Description of the process
7. Installation qualification protocol (main text)
8. Objective
9. Equipment verification
10. Equipment calibration requirements
11. Equipment maintenance requirements
12. Equipment cleaning requirements
13. Process specifications/operating parameters
14. Performance parameters
15. Quality parameters
16. Training

Installation Qualification Report

1. Title page
2. Identify the process, product, or equipment undergoing validation/qualification.
3. Identify the author of the protocol.
4. Abstract—briefly describe the intent of the protocol.
5. Protocol approval. Sign-off by Technology, Quality Assurance, and Manufacturing is required prior to performing the installation protocol.
6. Summary of results.
7. Objective.
8. Equipment verification.
9. Equipment calibration requirements.
10. Equipment maintenance requirements.

11. Equipment cleaning requirements.
12. Process specifications/operating parameters.
13. Performance parameters.
14. Training.

Performance Protocol

1. Title page.
2. Identify the process, product, or equipment undergoing validation/qualification.
3. Identify the author of the protocol.
4. Abstract—briefly describe the intent of the protocol.
5. Protocol approval. Technology, Quality Assurance, and Manufacturing approval is required prior to performing the performance protocol.
6. Introduction.
7. Objective.
8. Scope.
9. Background.
10. Performance qualification.
11. Procedure.
12. Performance parameters.
13. Inspection and test acceptance criteria.
14. Quality parameters (sampling).
15. Documentation.
16. List required SOPs (calibration, QA monitoring, production, maintenance requirements).
17. List required manuals, schematics.
18. List "as-built" drawing modification requirements, if applicable.
19. List spare parts requirements, if applicable.

Performance Protocol Report (Main Text)

1. Title page.
2. Identify the process, product, or equipment undergoing validation/qualification.
3. Identify the author of the protocol.

4. Abstract—briefly describe the intent of the protocol.
5. Validation package approval.
6. Sign-off by Technology, Quality Assurance, and Production.
7. Summary of results.
8. Objective.
9. Scope.
10. Documentation verification.
11. Calibration verification.
12. Performance verification/testing.
13. Conclusion.

Validation Package Approvals (General)

Installation qualification and performance protocols will be routed for approval. Area managers requesting revisions will document their requests. A protocol design review meeting will be initiated in cases of complex validations requiring input from all departments. Final approval of the validation package will be made after all documentation and appropriate personnel have completed training. Completed validations will be filed in Quality Assurance.

Equipment/Area Maintenance

All equipment must be fabricated in conformance with GMPs. Equipment should be free of sharp edges that could damage the product, should not generate excessive particulates while operating, and should not contaminate product with lubricants or by-products during operation. The equipment/area should be properly cleaned prior to the protocol run.

Revalidation

Revalidation may be necessary when

- There is a change in the actual process that may affect quality.

- There is an investigation of a negative trend in quality indicators.
- A change in the product design which affects the process.
- A process is transferred from one facility to another.
- The scope of application of the process has changed.

Protocol Execution

Prior to protocol execution, the following must occur to prevent compromising the study:

1. Equipment must be debugged and producing what appears to be acceptable product.
2. All equipment must be calibrated (as applicable).
3. Maintenance requirements during the run should be defined.

Retrospective Process Validation

In some cases a product may have been on the market without sufficient premarket process validation. In these cases, it may be possible to validate, in some measure, the adequacy of the process by examination of accumulated test data on the product and records of the manufacturing procedures used.

Retrospective validation can also be useful to augment initial premarket prospective validation for new products or changed processes. In such cases, preliminary prospective validation should have been sufficient to warrant product marketing. As additional data is gathered on production lots, such data can be used to build confidence in the adequacy of the process. Conversely, such data may indicate a declining confidence in the process and a commensurate need for corrective changes.

Test data may be useful only if the methods and results are adequately specific. As with prospective validation, it may be insufficient to assess the process solely on the basis of lot-by-lot conformance to specifications if test results are merely expressed in terms of pass/fail. Specific results, on the other hand, can be statistically analyzed and a determination can be made of what variance in data can be expected. It is important to maintain records that describe the operating characteristics of the process (e.g., time, temperature, humidity, and equipment settings). Whenever test data is used to demonstrate conformance to specifications, it is important that the test methodology be qualified to ensure that test results are objective and accurate.

Appendix H

Material Specification

MATERIAL SPECIFICATION 100-02

Vistanex LM-MH LC (Low Color) Polyisobutlylene Polymer

Rev.	DCR Date	Effective Date	Originator	Description
A	02-08-98	02-09-98	R. Bradley	Material specification
B	02-10-98	02-11-98	A. Sotnick	As per DCR 98-0002

Approved by: ______________________ Date: ____________

DESCRIPTION DETAILS

Vistanex LM-MH LC is a water-white to pale yellow, tacky, semi-solid polymer.

SPECIFICATIONS

Appearance: Water-white to pale yellow; Exxon Test Method #AMS 83-006
Penetration, MM @ 25(C: 15.4 -11.5; Exxon Test Method #AMS 210-10
Nonvolatile matter, WJ %: 97.0 min.; Exxon Test Method #AMS 82-003

APPLICABLE REFERENCE DOCUMENTS

Exxon "Vistanex LM Polyisobutylene, Low Color Grades"; Exxon Publication #102-1096-0101C dated October 1996; Exxon MSDS #84320000 dated April 13, 1996

RAW MATERIAL CODE

Vistanex LM-MH LC; Test RMC 90002

SAFETY AND HANDLING

Personnel Safety

Avoid eye and skin contact. Wear safety glasses with side shields, long sleeves, and chemical-resistant gloves. Avoid any contact with heat, open flames, or oxidizing materials. For eye contact flush with large amounts of clean water until irritation subsides. Then seek medical attention if irritation persists.

STORAGE REQUIREMENTS

Storage should be at ambient temperature. Electrostatic accumulation hazard should be minimized by proper grounding procedure during storage.

MATERIAL SAFETY DATA SHEETS

Exxon Chemical Company Polymers Group. MSDS No. 84320000

SAMPLING AND TESTING

Sampling

Per Quality Assurance Specification No. QS 700-90002

PACKAGING

Primary Package

A cylindrical paper fiber tube measuring 14½″ diameter × 24" height, with a close-fitting cap or the same material. The inside of the tube has a release agent to allow transfer of the contents out of the tube. The net content is 100# of product.

IDENTIFICATION MARKING

Exxon material name and lot number when received. BioDerm part number, lot number, and QC receiving inspections status when QC released.

VENDOR CERTIFICATION

A certificate of analysis will accompany each manufacturer's lot of product.

STATEMENTS AND NOTES

Safety and handling data (MSDS)

QUALITY CHARACTERISTICS

Chemical and physical properties and acceptable ranges:
Exxon Publication 102-1096 0101C dated Oct. 96
Characteristics, dimensions, color, mechanical requirements, general properties, and test requirement quality specification 700-90002.*

---

* See Appendix I.

Appendix I

Quality Specification

Company Name					Restricted Copy DO NOT COPY	
Quality Assurance Specification						
Subject:	**Vistanex LM-MH LC**				**QS No.**	**QS70060 02**
					Rev C	**Rev Date: 11/16/00**
					Effective:	**11/20/00**
Ref. Spec/ Procedure No.	**Cls. Def.**	**Unit Production Inspection**	**Characteristic Or Requirement**	**Inspection Method**	**Sampling Plan**	
					AQL Level	**A/R Level**
M6100002	**IV**	**100 lbs.**	**1.0 Documentation**	**Visual**	1 / lot	Present/ Within Spec
			1.1 Cert of analysis	Visual	1 / drum	0/1
			1.1.1Clear, water-white	Visual	1 / drum	0/1
			1.1.2 Penetration 11.5 to 15.4 mm	Exxon test	1 / drum	0/1
			1.1.3 Volatility 0.97% minimum	Exxon test	1 / drum	0/1
M6100002	**IV**	**100 lbs.**	**2.0 Material Identification**			
			2.1 Cert of analysis	Visual	1/ drum	0/1
			2.2 Lot no.	Visual	1/ drum	0/1
			2.3 Chemical name	Visual	1/ drum	0/1

Appendix J

Design Change Procedure

DOCUMENT CONTROL PROCEDURE

Rev.	DCR Date	Effective Date	Originator	Description
A	08-19-93		M.B. Robbins	Draft QA Policy
B	02-03-97	06-30-97	R. Bradley	Original release
C	06-25-97	06-30-97	J. Passero	DCR 97-0012
D	04-29-98	05-29-98	M. Teixeira	DCR 98-0064
E	08-12-98	08-14-98	R. Bradley	DCR 98-0148
F	09-14-99	10-08-99	M. Teixeira	DCR 99-0057

Approval Signature: ______________________ Date: ________________

1.0 PURPOSE

1.1 This procedure describes the system to be used for controlling quality system documents and data.

2.0 SCOPE

2.1 This procedure applies to all quality system documents identified within the quality system. It includes the initiation, review, approval, and distribution of new documents as well as changes to existing documents and obsolescence of documents (e.g., quality assurance policies, interim specifications, standard operating procedures, label text specifications, quality assurance specifications, material specifications, engineering drawings, forms, product specifications, technical files, device master records, quality plans, etc.).

3.0 DEFINITIONS

3.1 Approved document: An approved document is a document with approval from all required approving authorities.

3.2 Denied document: A denied document is a document not acceptable to an approving authority(s).

3.3 Withdrawn document: A withdrawn document is a document removed from the handling and approval cycle system (void).

3.4 Vendor or supplier verification: This is a response from a vendor or supplier defining its agreement to conform to the written requirements of a proposed specification/drawing. (This includes the acceptance of a purchase order.)

3.5 Specification/procedure books: These are controlled books assigned by Quality Assurance to departments/areas, which contain the current official approved copies of all assigned documents.

3.6 Master indexes: These lists, where practical, are maintained by Quality Assurance to identify the current revision of documents (e.g., QS index, SOP index, MS index, forms index, PD index, etc.). In most cases, the document number, title, revision level, and/or effectivity date are identified. The revision for each quality assurance policy (QAP) section is indicated in the table of contents. The effective date identified serves as both the revision and effectivity dates. These lists are updated as necessary in conjunction with the Notice of New Issue/Revision memo. (Note: Device master record revision = the date signed. Quality plan revision = revision letter. Technical file elements are per procedure.)

3.7 Distribution matrix: This is a matrix detailing the documents assigned to individual specification/procedure books or departments/areas.

3.8 Change history: This is the historical information for a document(s). The change history includes, at a minimum, a description of the change(s), identification of any affected documents, the signature and date of the approving individual, and the date the change becomes effective. The change history information for BioDerm documents is reflected on the documents and the completed DCR form.

3.10 Documentation change request (DCR) form: This is the document used to initiate changes to quality system documentation. Changes to quality system documentation include changes/revisions, new issues/additions, deviations, and obsolescence/deletions.

3.11 Approving authorities: Those individuals responsible for reviewing, approving, or denying a change to quality system documentation are the approving authorities.

4.0 RESPONSIBILITIES

Quality Assurance is responsible for controlling and maintaining quality system documents in accordance with this procedure, excluding engineering drawings.

Engineering is responsible for controlling and maintaining engineering drawings in accordance with this procedure.

4.2 All employees are responsible for adhering to the requirements of this procedure when submitting new or revised documents into the quality system.

5.0 REQUIRED EQUIPMENT

N/A

6.0 MATERIALS

N/A

7.0 RECORDS

Document change request form (DCR)

8.0 REFERENCE DOCUMENTS

Document indexes
SOP 100-003—Record retention procedure
SOP 100-008—Standard operating procedure
SOP 100-009—Quality assurance specifications
SOP 100-012—Label/labeling text specifications
SOP 100-013—Material specifications
SOP 100-017—Product specification procedure
SOP 100-024—Device master records
SOP 700-001—Technical file

Quality plans
Engineering drawings
Document distribution matrix

9.0 PROCEDURE

Making Changes to Quality System Documentation

The originator/requestor of a change to quality system documentation shall obtain a copy of a document change request (DCR) form from Quality Assurance.

The originator/requestor shall allocate the next available DCR number from the DCR log. (The DCR log is located in Quality Assurance.)

The originator/requestor shall complete the log for the DCR number (number, originator, date DCR initiated, and brief description).

As applicable, the originator/requestor will obtain an uncontrolled current copy of the quality system document that requires a change or revision from a controlled book.

The originator will make the necessary changes to the existing document by redlining the document to be changed. In extenuating circumstances, work to a red-line document will be permitted if all DCR form approvals have been given, while processing/editing the document occurs.

Documents should reference the DCR number in the header section of the document, if applicable, under "DESCRIPTION."

9.7 New documents or extensive changes/revisions to documents should be done on disk in the appropriate format.

9.8 When a change or revision affects more than one document, the originator/requestor shall identify responsibility for and/or submit changes for all affected documents.

9.9 Documentation change request DCR form:

The originator/requestor shall complete the DCR form as follows:

9.9.1 Record the request number, request date, and originator/requestor.
9.9.2 Identify documentation types affected (e.g., SOP, MS, QS, LT, etc.).
9.9.3 Identify request type (e.g., change/revision, new, deviation, obsolescence, etc.).
9.9.4 Identify effect code (if known).
9.9.5 Identify material disposition (if known).
9.9.6 Provide a complete and accurate reason for the requested change. (As applicable, include any reference to a nonconformance number, complaint number, audit observation number, etc.) Sufficient information is needed for approval authorities to enable them to have a complete understanding of the nature and impact of the request.
9.9.6.1 If introducing a new document, state the new documents application.
Example: This specification provides a process for assembling. . . .

9.9.7 The originator/requestor must provide a complete and accurate description of the requested change.
Example:
Change from: paragraph 3.3, maximum thickness 1.000 +/- .005″
Change to: paragraph 3.3, maximum thickness 1.000 +/- .002″
Note: Define and indicate the change completely and precisely.

9.9.7.1 A description of the required changes for complex/extensive documentation changes should be neatly printed or typed on a separate sheet of paper or on the back side of the DCR form. Attach the addendum sheet to the DCR Form.

9.9.8 Identify all known documents affected by indicating title and revision, and assigned to appropriate personnel.

9.9.9 The originator/requestor should acquire the signature of his or her department manager on the DCR form to indicate approval to proceed with the request and submit all required documentation to Quality Assurance.

9.9.10 DCR processing, review, approval, and distribution.

9.9.11 Quality Assurance will log in and assign a sequential request number for the DCR if not already done.

9.9.12 Quality Assurance will review all DCRs and associated documents for completeness and to ensure that no request for a change coming from other individuals or departments exists and/or will vary the intent of the original request.

9.9.13 Quality Assurance or designee will transcribe the document/document changes using a word processor.

9.9.14 Engineering is responsible for revising and controlling drawings. Engineering will revise specified drawings as needed and forward with the completed DCR form to Quality Assurance.

9.9.15 Quality Assurance or originator/requestor will route the DCR form along with the new or changed documents and all required attachments to the applicable approving departments as defined in Figure 1. The department head is considered the approving authority unless otherwise designated/delegated. (Note: Changes to quality system documents receive the same review and approval as the original document unless otherwise indicated. Approval designation is at the discretion of the Director of QA/RA.)

9.9.16 The approving authority is required to add additional documents, not identified, that may need to be revised as a result of the requested change. As an example, an engineering drawing change of a critical dimension may require changes in manufacturing SOPs, material specifications, QA specifications, label text specs, etc. The approving authority should add affected documents to the DCR form and assign the person responsible for making the appropriate changes. All additional changes should be made and submitted with the DCR form.

9.9.17 The approving authority approves documents by signing and dating the DCR form. Any minor or conditional changes to be made should be indicated by the approving authority. The approving authority denies documents by attaching a written explanation of the reasons for disapproval. The approving authority must provide written information to indicate any changes that would make the document acceptable (if appropriate).

9.9.18 Quality Assurance issues, withdraws, or returns the documents to the originator, based on DCR approval status.

	(QAP)	(SOP)	(MS)	(LT)	(PD)	(QS)	(IS)	(DEV)
Sales	x	*	-	*	-	-	*	*
Business Development	x	*	-	x	-	-	*	*
Technology	x	x	x	x	x	x	x	x
Quality Assurance/Regulatory Affairs	x	x	x	x	x	x	x	x
Manufacturing	x	x	x	*	x	-	x	x
Finance	x	*	x	x	x	x	*	*
Clinical Affairs	x	*	-	x	-	-	*	*
Engineering	x	*	*	-	x	x	*	*
Facilities	x	*	-	-	-	-	*	*
President/CEO	x	*	-	x	-	-	*	*

Note: Approval can always be delegated upward without written notification. QAP = Quality Assurance policy; SOP = standard operating procedure; MS = material specification; LT = label text specification; PD = product specification; QS = Quality Assurance specification; IS = interim specification; EDS = Engineering drawing specification; DEV = deviation; x = approval required; * = approval if department is affected (QA determines)

Figure 1 Necessary approving departments for certain forms.

9.9.19 The originator may review the denied DCRs with the appropriate approval authorities and may resubmit a revised DCR for consideration by documenting the necessary change(s) and recirculating the documents in accordance with this procedure.

SIGNIFICANCE OF APPROVAL

Approval of a DCR signifies that the designated approving authority has considered the best interests of the company and has determined that the approval of the DCR, including any deviations, will not adversely affect the safety and efficacy of any item or product.

DELEGATING APPROVAL AUTHORITY

To delegate approval authority, permanently or temporarily, forward a memo to Quality Assurance specifying the person(s) authorized to approve documents, the dates for which the authorization is valid, and any limitations (e.g., document types).

Quality Assurance will assign document numbers for new documents. Quality Assurance will print the document in the correct documentation form, route for approval, and distribute copies of the approved document as per the distribution matrix. Obsolete copies of all documents will be destroyed. The "obsolete" master document will be stamped obsolete and filed in Quality Assurance in accordance with the record retention procedure.

When desirable, quality system documents shall be color-coded to help rapidly identify them; the following colors will be used as follows:

Quality Assurance policy	Yellow/Melon
Standard operating procedures	White

Material specifications	Green
Product specifications	Blue
Interim specifications	Pink
Label text specs	White
Quality Assurance specs	Orange

Note: Only documents with a red or blue "Copy" stamp are considered controlled documents.

Communication of the issuance of a new document or a change to an existing document will be done by issuance of a "Notice of New Issue/Revision" memo to department heads/ specification/procedure book holders. This memo lists the documents affected and effective date and serves as notification of a change. Department heads are responsible for communicating the changes to their employees and providing training as necessary. The effective date of the document is also indicated on the document.

Note: Label/labeling text specifications may become effective prior to issuance of the Notice of New Issue/Revision Memo. (Only one master book is maintained in Q.A.) These documents will be reflected on the Notice of New Issue/Revision Memo at the time of next document update.

Finance is responsible for forwarding any copies of materials specifications, drawings, label text specifications, etc. that a supplier may need to meet purchase order or contract requirements. Finance will request vendor or supplier verification of the change. A vendor's or supplier's reply is expected within 4 to 6 weeks; nonreply is construed as agreement to the change, "as is."

At the time of distribution of any documents, Quality Assurance will update applicable document index(es).

10.0 SECURITY CONTROL CLASSIFICATION

10.1 All documents that make up the quality system are

considered "restricted" documents. Controlled copies of documents are issued by Quality Assurance and identified by a red or blue "Copy" stamp imprint. Controlled copies are to be made from the master document only.

10.2 Copies of documents for informational use or redlining may be made from controlled books. These copies are considered uncontrolled and may be stamped in red "Uncontrolled Copy."

Copies of documents for external distribution shall be stamped in red "Confidential Copy." External distribution of documents should be limited and authorized by department managers.

11.0 ELECTRONIC DOCUMENT CONTROL

11.1 All documents controlled by this procedure are stored via computer.

11.2 Entering new documents, deleting obsolete documents, and making revisions to current documents may only be accomplished by authorized personnel (primarily Quality Assurance; Engineering for drawings).

11.3 Electronic documents will be periodically backed up.

Index